The Allergy Problem

An account of the difficulties of allergic people which highlights the plight of those suffering from environmental intolerance and offers guidance to sufferers and their families.

The Allergy Problem

Why People Suffer and What Should be Done

by

Vicky Rippere
M.A., Ph.D., B.Sc., M.Phil.

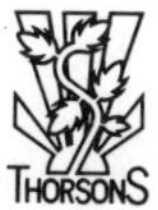

THORSONS PUBLISHERS LIMITED
Wellingborough, Northamptonshire

First Published 1983

© VICKY RIPPERE 1983

British Library Cataloguing in Publication Data

Rippere, Vicky
  The allergy problem.
    1. Allergy
    I. Title
  616.97 RC584

ISBN 0-7225-0867-0
ISBN 0-7225-0796-8 Pbk

Printed and bound in Great Britain

Contents

'It is my opinion that those who first called this disease 'sacred' were the sort of people we now call witch-doctors, faith healers, quacks and charlatans. These are exactly the people who pretend to be very pious and to be particularly wise. By invoking a divine element they were able to screen their own failure to give suitable treatment and so called this a 'sacred' malady to conceal their ignorance of its nature.'

Hippocrates, *The Sacred Disease* [1]

. . . we ought to ask ourselves . . . how much we really know about the problems of living to which certain chronic illness gives rise.

Anselm L. Strauss *Chronic Illness and the Quality of Life* [2]

This book is also dedicated to all patients who have ever been called neurotic, hypochondriacal, hysterical, or starved for attention, while actually suffering from environmentally induced illness.[3]

Foreword

Readers of this book who are unfamiliar with clinical ecology may conclude that the premise on which it is based, that allergic reactions to foods and/or environmental chemicals can take the form of a wide variety of physical and mental conditions, is too questionable to merit the serious attention of such a highly qualified clinical psychologist as Dr Rippere. 'Certainly,' such readers will think, 'medicine is so scientific and progressive that if clinical ecology really were effective it would have been quickly adopted into the standard medical armamentarium.' While some medical innovations are quickly accepted – so quickly in fact, that patients are frequently harmed by failure of doctors to recognize their limitations and hazards – other new ideas languish unrecognized for long periods of time.

English doctors failed for decades to adopt the use of the stethoscope in the nineteenth century because not only was it an invention of the then-hated French but its use was considered undignified for physicians. In 1911, some forty-five years before the development of polio vaccine, Sister Elizabeth Kenny discovered a method for treating that dread disease that was much less painful for the patient and produced more complete recoveries than the treatment then in use. Unable to get acceptance of her ideas in her native Australia she travelled to London and eventually to America. Finally, some American doctors listened to her and concluded she was right. Only then, thirty years after she originated it, was the Kenny method widely adopted. She had been right all along, but more than a generation of polio sufferers had to pay the price in pain and crippling for the refusal of doctors to assess properly her contribution.

There are many other examples of belated recognition of new ideas in medicine, so that the fact that clinical ecology is still not accepted by conventional medicine, or at best is considered 'controversial', is not proof that it deserves its present status.

The reason we are likely to think of medicine as being so receptive to innovation is that we constantly hear of exciting new developments such as heart transplants, intensive care units, CAT scanners, and wondrous new drugs. But innovations such as these almost invariably involve expensive new surgical techniques and profitable developments in either high technology or patented medications. Given this situation, a method of treating illness that simply calls for avoiding certain foods or chemical exposures is likely to be trampled upon in the race for prestige and profits, even if the method was first developed by a highly respected physician such as Dr Herbert Rinkel.

The basic principles of clinical ecology are quite simple. When one is allergic to a food eaten only occasionally, the reaction to that food – whether a skin rash, digestive upset, headache, or whatever – will be recognized by the person, who will learn to avoid that food. With foods eaten every day or so, however, (which also are likely to be ones eaten since childhood before a reaction could be recognized) the body tries to *adapt* to them just as to any other stress. As long as the adaptation holds, the person will be in generally good health and, if allergy had been recognized in childhood the person would be described as having 'outgrown' it. But for some people the stress caused by the allergy is too great to permit successful adaptation, while others may have their adaptation eventually break down with resultant physical and/or mental symptoms.

Treatment for food allergy requires that the guilty foods be detected and avoided. When this is done improvement quickly follows. The majority of food sensitivities are not *fixed* (i.e permanent) but are *cyclical*, meaning that after a period of complete avoidance of perhaps several months the food can then be eaten safely providing it is not eaten too frequently, say, more often than once every four days.

Readers may be surprised to find references in this book to

food addiction. We all know that people can become addicted to heroin or barbiturates, but addiction to milk or oranges or bread? What happens, according to clinical ecologists, is that the body, in the process of trying to adapt to the stress caused by the guilty substances, is altered biochemically, including increased adrenaline output. The person then gets used to this altered state caused by eating the allergenic foods, and comes to define it as normal. Eating these foods gives the person an internal biochemical 'fix' so that he/she feels better afterwards. Avoiding the guilty foods stops the process, which can result in producing actual withdrawal symptoms.

After four or five days of complete avoidance of a food the body loses its adaptation to it so that if the food is then eaten the person will ordinarily get a reaction to it soon enough afterwards to indicate that the food is allergenic for that person. A rotation diet, in which a variety of foods are eaten, but no single food more often than once every four days, thus can be both a means of detecting food sensitivities and a way of preventing new sensitivities from developing as a result of too-frequent consumption of a food.

Although food has been emphasized here, people can also be affected by environmental chemicals, which include such common items as household detergents, plastics, synthetic fabrics, cosmetic and toiletry items, petrol and exhaust fumes, and insecticides whether from spray cans or as residues – even in officially approved amounts – on foods. Taking all this into account we can see how conditions caused by allergy can be viewed as ecological illness.

Dr Rippere describes her own difficulties with what she eventually learned was allergy. Most proponents of clinical ecology, both medical and lay people (including myself), are individuals who suffered from various conditions caused by allergy and saw them corrected by allergen detection and appropriate avoidance. The idea that allergic reactions are all in the mind is simply untenable. Randolph and Mackarness and others have done blind and double-blind studies noting patients' reactions to tube-fed food and found that responses were to the actual substances administered. Even when patients were misled as to the type of food being given by tube the reaction, or lack of it, was to the food and not to what the patient believed it to be. There is no sound scientific basis to justify statements of conventional doctors that allergic reactions or improvements caused by changes in diet are 'only psychological' or are due to the 'placebo effect', etc.

Some critics of this study, particularly in view of Dr Rippere's revelation of her personal experience with clinical ecology, conceivably could argue that it has made her unduly biased in favour of the field and keeps her from being objective about it as a researcher. A careful reading of this study will show that this is not the case. If knowing from experience or academic knowledge what types of questions to ask on a questionnaire is a basis for disqualifying a study, then practically all studies in psychology and sociology should be considered invalid. On the contrary, some of our most valuable contributions in the behavioural sciences have come from a research method known as participant observation, in which a researcher immerses himself or herself in a certain milieu and reports on it from the standpoint of one from the outside who has experienced it from the inside.

The sample in the study is not a random cross-section of the British population, nor is it claimed to be. As data on its composition show, it is unrepresentative in including a disproportionate number from the higher social classes and none from the lowest classes. Given the means used to obtain respondents and the nature of the questionnaire, this is probably unavoidable. Practically always, samples in the behavioural sciences wind up with under-representation from those at the lower social levels. but the very fact of sample bias suggests certain conclusions. If relatively well-off people above average in social status can have as much difficulty as they report here in coping with allergy and relating to their friends and physicians, how much more difficult it must be for people in the lower classes not adequately represented in this study, who do not possess as many advantages.

The experiences of the respondents are sobering. We see grown men and women, many of them professionals, responsible members of their respective communities, being treated with arrogance and condescension by doctors and nurses ignorant of their true condition. Their painfully obtained knowledge about things that affect them is discounted and ridiculed by those who should be helping them. It is amazing how many respondents use the words 'sceptical' or 'scepticism' in their comments in describing the reactions of others to their problems. Many of them conclude they must deceive their physicians about their allergies and the means they are using to deal with them in order to maintain a viable relationship that might be needed for other medical problems.

The study also brings out the obstacles allergy sufferers have to overcome in coping with their allergies on a day-to-day basis. The difficulties in getting suitable food (without milk or wheat, for example) are considerable, but the complications are greatly increased when one is eating away from home. Friends, whom one would like to think would give help and understanding, sometimes create serious problems. The idea that a person's friends would deliberately include a food to which the person was sensitive in a meal they were giving him is appalling, and yet this was reported. One is reminded of the saying that with friends like those a person doesn't need enemies.

More commonly, the problems result from ignorance and inability to comprehend what allergy is really all about. Even here, though, part of the cause must be ascribed to the medical profession which, as a result of its refusal to entertain new ideas about allergy, perpetuates ignorance by lay people. After all, if the doctors don't believe in it, how can one expect a friend or neighbour to? Yet the respondents found lay people more understanding than medical professionals.

Dr Rippere's respondents made me aware of how in one way I have been insulated from the tendency of friends not to accept the validity of the allergic person's condition and the means necessary to cope with it. My friends know I have written a book about allergy, and even if they haven't read it, simply its existence tends to authenticate any statement I might make about foods I can or cannot have. The typical allergy sufferer does not have this advantage and so is more likely to encounter disbelief and failure to be taken seriously.

Some individuals, particularly physicians, might have reservations about Dr Rippere's proposal that people with allergy problems be helped by professionals other than MDs. Is she advocating the practice of medicine without a licence? To answer this question let us ask just what is really involved in the practice of medicine. Clearly, the use of invasive procedures for diagnosis and treatment, and the supervision of patients who have hazardous physical or mental reactions to foods to which they are allergic are matters for physicians. But certainly not every statement made by one person to another about foods and possible consequences of eating them can be considered the practice of medicine. If a person mentions to a neighbour that he has trouble getting to sleep and the neighbour suggests avoiding coffee one would not expect the neighbour to be charged with the practice of medicine. People chat with each other all the time about things they eat and their possible effects. Advertisements on commercial radio and television and in the printed media regularly tell us to eat or not eat certain foods for a variety of reasons including health and attitudes, and yet this is not considered the practice of medicine.

Somewhere between the two extremes of the clearly medical on the one hand and just conversation about food on the other is an area where responsible non-MD professionals could perform a valuable service by giving information to individuals to aid them in assessing the effects that particular foods may have upon them. Furthermore, many of these effects are psychological, which is the traditional and legitimate domain of the behavioural sciences. Dr Rippere uses the term behavioural ecology to refer to the area of the influence of foods and other factors in the environment upon emotions and mental functioning. It seems completely appropriate for it to be a part of psychology. I do not believe that psychologists, social workers, and similar professionals are really interested in practising medicine, but I can understand how they would want to be able to make useful information available to their clients. I am sure the clients would want this also and would greatly benefit from it.

After all, it is the person afflicted with food sensitivities that we need to keep in mind. Gilbert and Sullivan made the case that the policeman's lot is not a happy one. Now, Dr Rippere's study shows that neither is that of the allergy sufferer. While some of the unpleasantness is caused by the condition itself and the limitations in diet and lifestyle that it may impose, many difficulties are attributable to ignorance and thoughtlessness of other people, both medical and lay, and consequently are susceptible to amelioration through greater knowledge of the type that this book seeks to impart.

ROBERT FORMAN PHD
Professor of Sociology
The University of Toledo
Toledo, Ohio, U.S.A.

Introduction

This book is about the problems that people who react adversely to common factors in our environment – foods, chemicals, fumes, dust, animals, pollens, smoke, drugs, and the like – encounter in their efforts to live ordinary lives in the community. My main thesis is that a moderate to severe degree of intolerance to environmental factors may constitute a serious social handicap, which is most often overlooked or discounted by outsiders. This conclusion results from the findings of a study of the experiences and special problems of a group of eighty five people who suffer from one or more of the many conditions that may be grouped under the general heading of environmental intolerance. The aim of the book is to present my findings in some detail.

The study, which was carried out in 1979-80 with the help of several self-help and special-interest groups, was intended to collect descriptive data about the typical hazards of possessing an allergic or hypersensitive constitution whilst inhabiting an environment in which the sorts of physical stimuli most likely to provoke symptoms are either intermittently or constantly present. Thus the study dealt with the effects of allergic reactivity rather than with the causes of the condition. At the present time, the underlying biological mechanisms responsible for causing allergic reactions are undergoing intensive study in major research centres all over the world. But the effects of allergy, intolerance, and hypersensitivity upon the social and psychological functioning of people whose bodies are so unfortunate as to house these scientifically fascinating anomalies remain virtually unknown. From the important, but generally undervalued, point of view of the sufferer, the effects of the disorder – for instance the fact that it may virtually preclude normal social life – are more salient and poignant than the fact, however indubitable, that it arises from the degranulation of mast cells when antigen and antibody collide.

Because the effects of being an allergic person have hitherto been widely ignored as topics for serious concern, it may be well to set forth some of my reasons for believing that they are worthy of attention. The first reason is that unless more people know about them, nothing much is likely to be done to improve the lot of sufferers. My findings suggest that there is a very real and widespread need, not only for better services for the afflicted but also for more sympathetic medical and public attitudes to them. These needs seem unlikely to be met unless their existence is recognized. And a second reason for wishing to draw attention to the unfortunate social effects of allergy and environmental intolerance is that unless something is done about it, the situation is likely to get worse. As our physical environment and food supply become more contaminated with the residues of so-called technological progress, people who develop symptoms upon exposure to these residues, whether they be chemical additives or food substances such as wheat flour, sugar, milk powder, egg, or whatever, will find it progressively harder to avoid them. More people will also become affected. Unless the situation of sufferers improves, more and more people will find themselves ill, misunderstood, ostracized, largely unable to obtain needed help through official channels, and increasingly at a disadvantage in social situations.

At the present time, there appears to be a tremendous amount of prejudice against people with ecological disorders. As is shown in this book, other people's intolerance of them for being different is as grievous an affliction as their own biological intolerance of the allergens which singles them out from the mass of people who can come into contact with these substances without becoming ill. An example will illustrate this prejudice in action.

In the spring of 1981, I presented the preliminary results of the survey to the inaugural conference of the Society for

Environmental Therapy at Oxford[1]. After my lecture, many sufferers and practitioners in the audience expressed their appreciation of the presentation. One long-suffering lady came up to thank me on behalf of fellow victims 'for putting our point of view across'. A few weeks later, another very different reaction came my way. The writer expressed harsh criticism of the paper. He dismissed it as 'completely uncritical' – presumably since I had taken my respondents' reports at face value instead of discounting what they had said, rejected my sample as invalid because in addition to people suffering from true allergies it 'probably contained anorexics, agoraphobics, and just plain nutters', and criticized my respondents as irresponsible because 'patients who established their own diagnoses have fools for physicians'. Now the point of my paper had been that many sufferers have to work out the connections between their symptoms and the environmental factors provoking them all by themselves because they cannot get the help they need from their doctors, and that what they tend to get from them instead of the help they need is a lot of psychiatric name-calling, inappropriate referrals for fruitless investigations, and palliative treatment with drugs that don't work. I described one of their most outstanding problems as the fact that they are so often rejected completely out of hand as 'nutters' by attitudinizing people – such as the critic himself – who not only do not understand what is going on with them but also apparently cannot be bothered to find out. The virulence and sheer inconsequentiality of this supposedly scientific opinion of my paper exemplify precisely the sort of negative social stereotyping I was trying to criticize in it. The criticism adds weight to my argument rather than detracting from it.

My argument is, then, that these sorts of cruel and mindless negative attitudes constitute a major burden which allergic and hypersensitive people, already laden with the practical difficulties they encounter in their commerce with the physical environment, get lumbered with in their everyday dealings with the social milieu. It is hard enough to try to avoid contact with common substances of which others may not even be aware; it is hard, too, if one's efforts are unsuccessful, because then one develops symptoms. But if on top of all this hardship one also has to contend with being regarded as a social freak, it is really all a bit much and the social stigma, at least, is quite unnecessary. Hardest of all, perhaps, is the fact that doctors and other helping professionals seem to be the worst offenders in thus adding insult to injury.

In thinking about the suffering caused by human disease, we need to distinguish between different orders of problem. Wing's taxonomy of the handicaps of people suffering from schizophrenia[2] makes the useful distinction between primary, secondary and tertiary handicaps. These concepts are useful in the present context:

Primary handicaps are those arising from the biology of the illness and include symptoms and difficulties which follow immediately from them.

Secondary handicaps are those arising from changes in the person's social relationships as a function of other people's perception of him as a sufferer from his primary handicaps as well as those resulting from changes in his perception of himself as a function of both of these factors.

Tertiary handicaps include pre-existing social disadvantages such as poor education, work skills, employment record, poverty, unemployment, poor housing and living conditions and the like, which may be related to the person's other difficulties but which could also exist independently of them. In general these sorts of factors tend to complicate the management of any chronic illness.

Let us now apply these notions to the people who suffer from some form of environmental intolerance.

For allergic and hypersensitive people, primary handicaps may be of two main types. First of all there are the problems arising from symptoms that occur when the person is exposed to his allergens. But in addition to these more immediate effects of the biological condition itself, there are also a whole host of other problems arising from that person's efforts to identify the causes of the symptoms and thereafter to prevent their occurrence by avoiding the precipitants or enhancing the body's ability to tolerate unavoidable exposure.

Both the symptoms themselves and the regimen which the person must adopt in order to avoid them contribute to the formation of secondary handicaps. For some victims, the strategies and tactics they find they have to engage in to remain well are responsible for more social and psychological disadvantage than are the symptoms themselves. With perseverance and planning, it is possible for some sufferers to prevent the appearance of symptoms, by means of strict adherence to their self-management regimen. But the cost of doing so may be heavy – loss of social opportunities, multiple misunderstandings, and a deviant social identity.

These secondary hazards, in addition to the primary biological ones, may be responsible for tertiary problems. These may take the form of reducing earning capacity through limitations on the person's ability to work, with a consequently lowered standard of living, social isolation, and general impoverishment of life chances. As a result of these losses, the sufferer is likely to come to possess fewer of the material resources which are necessary to facilitate avoidance of allergens and the orginal problem may be compounded. Such vicious circles are not uncommon in sufferers' reports of their experiences.

Amongst these vicious circles, perhaps none is more unfortunate nor more unnecessary than the exacerbation of sufferers' difficulties that so often seems to result from their attempts to obtain medical help. Medical care can be hazardous to the health of the allergic or hypersensitive individual for a number of different reasons, an important one being that so many are unable to obtain the sort of help they need. In this country, clinical ecologists are in short supply and those few who practise this new speciality are not accessible to the great mass of the afflicted public, either for geographical or for financial reasons. And even when clinical ecology facilities are available, prospective patients may not be able to obtain a referral from their GP. One survey respondent, for example, reported that he had asked his GP for a letter to a local practitioner. His lay NHS-based therapist also wrote to the GP making the same request. But, the respondent reported, the GP 'dismissed the idea as ridiculous'. Other respondents described attending their clinical ecologist or alternative practitioner without the GP's knowledge – and with some trepidation in case he found out. Only two respondents in the entire eighty five said that their GP had been able to recognize the true nature of their condition and to diagnose it himself without the aid of a specialist. Many others described having been sent for orthodox medical investigations of varying degrees of obnoxiousness, only to be told when all the results had come back that nothing wrong had been found so that, therefore, no treatment could be offered. Meanwhile, in the absence of appropriate help, their suffering merely continued.

A second reason why medical care can damage the health of the allergic and hypersensitive is that the investigations to which they may be submitted can involve exposure to their allergens, often when they are in a hypersensitive, fasting state. Two respondents described having had adverse reactions to the 'fatty meal' mixture consumed for cholecystograms and another to the glucose consumed for a glucose tolerance test.[3] Another developed a rash from the paste used to apply EEG electrodes to the scalp. In the first three cases, each patient, recognizing the exposure hazard, had tried to alert staff to the imminence of an adverse reaction and in all cases their understandable concern was dismissed as unfounded, with depressingly predictable results. One of the reactions was reported to have required treatment from the patient's GP.

A third reason is that treatment itself may entail exposure to sufferers' idiosyncratically dangerous substances. Not only are drugs, antibiotics, the binder in tablets, and anaesthetics potentially hazardous to some allergic individuals, but also, more basically, hospital food and water may cause some of them to develop symptoms and these are less likely than drug reactions to be attributed to the correct source. Many respondents mentioned having had adverse reactions to medications that they were given, and quite a few expressed concern about whether they would be able to eat anything if they had to be admitted to hospital. One said that she was asked about her allergies upon admission but then was served dishes containing them at almost every meal.

Fourth, in addition to adverse reactions to physical stimuli encountered in medical settings, allergic and hypersensitive people are also at particular risk of unsympathetic handling by medical and paramedical staff. Undoubtedly many non-allergic people will be able to identify with the plight of the typical sufferer from masked allergy who, upon developing symptoms that do not yield to simple commonsense measures, consults the doctor in the hope of being given understanding, useful advice and effective help, only to be dismissed with admonition that 'it's just your nerves/your age/your attitude', or some other similar brush-off. It is not for nothing that ours has been described as the 'age of psychogenic dismissal'.[4] The survey results suggest that possibly the one sort of disorder that is more prone than endocrine disease to attract a swarm of erroneous functional psychiatric attributions is the ecological disorder, particularly if it is not characterized by obvious skin lesions or acute respiratory distress. If the victim persists in complaining, and expresses concern that the symptoms are worsening rather than yielding to palliative treatment – often in form of tranquillizers, his distress is then laid at the door of the effects which the toxic condition, unrecognized and untreated, has created in its wake. Thus he is told that the reason for the symptoms is *because* he is depressed or upset or whatever, and, if this advice doesn't relieve the symptoms, because he needs an excuse for constant attention-seeking. This sort of 'explanation' is very convenient for the professional 'helper' who offers it, because it virtually ensures the prompt disappearance of all but the most thick-skinned sufferer from the surgery or clinic. But for the sufferer, such a perversely tautologous put-down can be both extremely painful and humiliating. To those who have not experienced a similar situation, my depiction may seem like a caricature. Those who have had the misfortune to be expected to find such elucidations either illuminating or reassuring, however, will recognize in it the essence of their predicament.

The name of the game – and we need to call it by its name – is 'Blame the Victim'.[5] Its dynamics include the prevalent, if now tottering, myths of medical omniscience and omnipotence and the threat to this myth which the patient's intractable suffering comprises. No doctor with any humane pretensions likes to be confronted by symptoms that continue despite his persistent efforts to banish them and he vents his frustration upon the patient whose recalcitrant afflictions have evoked it. But the myth that the doctor can always make it better is not the only element in the drama. Blaming the victim takes place against the background of contemporary cultural fashions in disease.[6] There are many patients whose illness is equally unyielding in the face of medical intervention but who manage to avoid being cast in the role of scapegoat for the professional's inability to understand the cause or to effect a radical cure. But these illnesses, the tragic degenerative diseases of childhood foremost amongst them – muscular dystrophy, cystic fibrosis, and the like – have a certain stark public respectability, which is reflected in the existence of influential national organizations aimed at stimulating public concern and promoting research.

Everyone has seen the hoarding posters of stricken youngsters gazing wistfully from their wheelchairs and crutches. But although there are now patient-interest organizations for the allergic, who could imagine a poster depicting a middle-aged housewife vomiting convulsively in the throes of a bad migraine or a hyperactive toddler tearing the house apart after scoffing a roll of multicoloured sweeties? I am not for a moment decrying the posters of stricken children, who need all the help, acceptance and public support that they – and their desperate parents — can get. But it is nonetheless clear that there are public fashions in acceptable diseases and that allergy, hypersensitivity and environmental intolerance, which affect a much greater proportion of the population than the relatively rare degenerative diseases on the posters, attract public attention, sympathy and support in no proportion to their prevalence.

The blaming of allergic and hypersensitive people for having symptoms that do not conform to a textbook organic disease stereotype and do not get better when treated as functional with allopathic remedies does not end with dismissive psycho-diagnoses. The victims are regarded as culpable whatever they do. Those who seek help outside the system have recently been described in the correspondence columns of the *British Medical Journal* as resorting to cranks.[7] And, as we saw in the critique of my conference paper mentioned earlier, those who find they must resort to self-help because outside help has not been forthcoming or fruitful, may be denounced as irresponsible fools for taking into their own hands matters that are regarded as properly only the concern of doctors. In such cases, where the critic is speaking of such patients in the abstract, personal frustration at his own inability to help them cannot be a factor. It is these sorts of gratuitous and impersonal condemnations that reveal the victim-bashing syndrome as a generalized medical stance. This indiscriminate castigation of sick people who are only trying to get better and who must depart from orthodox methods because orthodoxy has abdicated responsibility for their care is a sorry commentary on medical expertise in the last quarter of the twentieth century.

Although doctors and paramedical staff are the strongest contenders in the Olympics of blame, they are by no means the only contestants in the field. At the present time, the knowledgeability, tolerance and sympathy of the general public also leave much to be desired. But in contrast to the conspicuous foot-dragging of medical orthodoxy, the general public's level of awareness of the condition seems to be proceeding by leaps and bounds. Hardly a month goes by without an article on food allergy or household toxicology appearing in one of the leading popular magazines. The problem with the new interest in allergy amongst the public, however, is that as usual readers seem to be more interested in allergic phenomena with possible relevance to their own personal case than, as yet, in the day-to-day secondary problems of their unfortunate fellows who manifest these phenomena. And, as yet, apart from a few concessions in public places to those who react adversely to smoke, the spreading public awareness does not seem to have been translated into the sort of practical action – such as provision of plain, junk-free food in British Rail catering facilities, labelled menus in restaurants, full explicit packet labelling, and the automatic provision of self-catering facilities at residential conferences, for example – that would make the lives of sufferers considerably less difficult and limited.

Still, the greatest problems undoubtedly remain in the medical sphere, where patients lack the degree of choice that is normally available to them in the outside world. If they go travelling, inconvenient and cumbersome as it may be, they are free to take their own food supplies along. If eating out, they can probably manage to select plain and safe fare from the menu and if they require information about ingredients, the management of most reputable establishments will bend over backwards to be of assistance once they appreciate the nature of the customer's difficulties. But in hospital, choice is severely limited and vital information is difficult to obtain. Requests for special consideration are likely to be met with being regarded as 'difficult', 'hypochondriacal' or 'manipulative', and staff response is more likely to be withdrawal than co-operation, [8] largely because if staff fail to understand the nature of the patient's very real problem they are unable to recognize the medical legitimacy of his requests and concern.

While there is no guarantee that better understanding on the part of doctors, paramedical staff and the general public will lead to improvements in the situation of sufferers from the many and varied disorders comprising environmental intolerance, it is practically a foregone conclusion that unless the community at large becomes more knowledgeable about and sympathetic towards the everyday problems of allergic and hypersensitive people, these problems are likely to continue. It is my hope that this account of the difficulties will help make it possible for the non-allergic reader to understand his allergic neighbour better, for the non-allergic hostess to show consideration for the welfare of her allergic guests, for the non-allergic managers of hotels, restaurants, airlines and the like to cater for the special needs of their allergic guests and passengers, and for those who make public-policy decisions at national, regional and local levels to appreciate the nature of the many problems and needs which the system at present sadly neglects to meet. Perhaps more important, I hope that this book will also help make it possible for those working in the field who will have to implement the new policies and practices that must be developed to appreciate the position in which having an allergic constitution places the sufferer.

1.

Food Allergy: A personal account

The results of the survey will probably be more meaningful to readers who do not themselves suffer from allergy or hypersensitivity if we begin with a concrete example, examined in some detail. My own case will serve this purpose.

Ever since I can remember, I have always had problems with foods. Although I was considered a healthy child, I often felt nauseous, vomited more than most kids I knew, and was well aware what a headache was before I started school. At home I was regarded as 'having a thing' about certain foods – eggs, milk and cooked breakfast cereals in particular. Breakfast was the worst meal of the day, especially in winter, when my mother would serve us bowls of steamy wheaten porridge, which I always felt would be more suitable for laying pavements with than for human consumption. I would feel sick on the way to school and would then sit all morning in the classroom, more attentive to the unpleasant heavy lump inside me than to the mysteries of short division. At mid-morning break, I refused to drink the lukewarm, waxy milk unless I could disguise the taste with chocolate syrup brought from home, but I still felt bad after I'd got it down. My difficulties were generally attributed to 'being difficult' and nothing official, like asking the doctor, was done about them, except to punish me from time to time for refusing to consume what was set before me. I felt like a freak because everyone else I knew seemed to *like* milk.

Once, after gagging on some eggs, I dug my heels in and

wouldn't eat them any more and there was nothing anyone could do to make me. Then one lunchtime at school I arrived at the canteen to discover that the menu for the day was scrambled eggs. I told the nice supply teacher who was taking our class that day that I couldn't eat eggs without being sick. 'Oh, my daughter is allergic to eggs, too,' she said, and wrote a note to the canteen ladies explaining my predicament. They were terribly nice about it and gave me soup and sandwiches instead. That was the first time I heard the word 'allergic'. I wasn't sure what it meant exactly, but from the context it seemed to mean awkward people like me who couldn't eat ordinary things like everyone else did. I was about eight or nine at the time.

The first migraine I can place a definite date on occurred on my tenth birthday. For a treat, my parents took us – my brother, sister and me – to the Catskill Game Farm, a sort of private open zoo with tame animals wandering about. After a marvellous day of molesting the livestock and making the usual nuisance of ourselves, we had hamburgers and french fries at a roadside café on the way home. Back on the road, I soon developed a blinding headache and had to ask my father to stop the car several times so I could vomit. That headache wasn't the first, nor was it to be the last, but it was nearly another twenty years before I had a name for it. Meanwhile, my tendency to get so ill after eating things that the others could just enjoy confirmed my growing suspicion that I must be very peculiar indeed.

Over the years, the headaches persisted. Many pleasant days ended in nausea, flashing lights and a pounding head. Gradually I began to avoid the foods that seemed to detonate this chain of events – fatty and fried things, liver sausage, bacon, elaborate sauces, red wine. There were probably a great many more things disagreeing with me even then, but they were more subtle about it and I couldn't pinpoint them with any certainty. At home, no one made a fuss about my occasional episodes of turning pale, retiring to the dark, and vomiting till all I was fit for was sleep. My parents weren't great ones for consulting doctors. Sometimes my mother was forced to when her asthma got very bad, and my father had to have treatment once for an ulcer. But, generally speaking, as a family we enjoyed reasonably good health and didn't have much to do with the medical profession. Any fuss that was made centred on my persistent reluctance to consume milk, eggs, bread and cereals, since they only made me feel ill but didn't produce headaches. Whatever was wrong with me obviously wasn't fatal, since it had been going on for years and I was more or less OK between episodes. And my affliction, also obviously, wasn't food poisoning, because the others ate the same food without getting sick.

During my first two years at university, I lived in a hall of residence, where meals were provided. There it wasn't always possible to rule out food poisoning. Not infrequently, when I spent the evenings running up and down the corridor to the loo until the early hours of the morning, I had a lot of company. As my headaches got worse my food choice became increasingly defensive. I found that the less the canteen staff had done to prepare something, the less likely it seemed to make me ill. Accordingly, I lived on grapefruit, bananas, apples, pears, oranges, boiled eggs, cottage cheese, yoghurt, cheese and biscuits, carrot and celery sticks, plain salads with cheese or cold meat, and the cakes and pastry which they got from a local bakery. I surprised myself by coming to tolerate eggs, which I had never thought I'd be able to stand. But eating them was better than missing a meal, which by then I had discovered also gave me a headache. At times I felt trapped by my body and circumstances. There were periods when, no matter what I did or didn't do, it would make me sick. Life became unpredictable, since even with all my spreading dietary restrictions, something would still catch up with me from time to time and at the last minute I'd find myself throwing up again when I should have been going out. Being at the mercy of my erratic body in this way was demoralizing.

After two years of this regimen, my growing intolerance of institutional cooking came to dictate my choice of accommodation. The headaches, diarrhoea and general malaise were starting to interfere with my studies and I also felt sure I was developing vitamin deficiencies into the bargain. I prevailed upon my father to allow me to live off campus, where I could do my own cooking, during my third year. He saw my point and supported my application for a place in a new self-catering unit that the college was opening. During my third year, I found I had considerably fewer headaches and less general ill-health than during the past two years. But if I ate in restaurants or at parties, my deviations would catch up with me.

Thereafter, being able to do my own catering assumed increasingly higher priority in my personal scheme of things. I resisted accepting this socially inconvenient necessity as long as possible, but over the years I had so many occasions to discover the unwelcome truth of the fact that I was less likely than others to serve me foods that disagreed that I was finally forced to admit that the conclusion was inescapable.

During the summer between my third and fourth year at university, I went to the Continent with the intention of travelling for a month, studying for six weeks at the Sorbonne, and resuming my travels until September, when the plane would return to New York. After the first month, I reluctantly added travelling to the growing list of events that I didn't seem able to tolerate. At the Sorbonne I was offered accommodation with a local family, which undoubtedly would have been excellent for my French, but it would have involved an intolerable degree of uncertainty about my diet and a consequent risk to my studies. My French wasn't up to the task of explaining my difficulties and, being unfamiliar with the culture, I didn't know whether people would understand them even if I had had the words to explain. So instead, I moved into a tiny *chambre de bonne* on the top floor of a block near St Lazare and for the six weeks prepared most of my meals in the room with only a knife, a chopping board and a small immersion heater. I found one restaurant where the cooked food didn't seem to upset me, so I was able to supplement the cold sandwiches, boiled eggs, cheese, raw vegetables and fresh fruit that I lived on otherwise. When the course finished, I couldn't face another round of travelling and constant headaches, so I decided to remain in Paris until it was time to return home. I found another *chambre*, this time with the luxury of an electric hotplate, on which I learnt to make onion soup. During the day, I worked on my dissertation in one of the libraries and remained well, with the exception of a week-long attack of something like dysentery after eating a tin of some unnameable French savoury.

In my final year I shared a flat. Neither my flatmate nor I had much money, but by dint of careful bargain-hunting we evolved a reasonably sensible, if monotonous, diet based on minced beef, a weekly chicken, eggs, processed cheese, pasta, rye bread, fruit and vegetables, with occasional self-indulgent gallons of ice-cream. We'd have cheeseburgers for breakfast, cheeseburgers for lunch, and a proper cooked meal in the evening. There was always plenty of fruit and raw vegetables to nibble; biscuits and other baked goods weren't safe against the mice. At the end of the year, I expected that I'd never wish to see – let alone eat – another cheeseburger again in my life, but was surprised to find that I could no longer imagine eating anything else for breakfast. I was, of course, by this time well and truly addicted to all my dietary staples — wheat and rye, milk and cheese, beef, tomatoes, lettuce, eggs and chicken, not to mention coffee, which I drank, black, by the gallon, but since I had no concept of food addiction, I was only happy to have found a diet that actually seemed to like me. After years of metabolic persecution, it was a welcome change.

The following year I developed my addictive lifestyle in a small flat in Cambridge, Massachusetts, while I studied for a Master's degree at Harvard. Because the flat lacked a fridge, and because my busy timetable only allowed for twice-weekly food shopping, I came to rely on tinned meat savouries — corned beef and corned-beef hash, meatballs, spam and the like — that didn't require refrigeration. On weekends I could break the monotony with a fresh or frozen chicken quarter, minced lamb, or some fish, but during the week, week in and week out, I would have eggs and last night's leftovers for breakfast, a hot pastrami sandwich on rye with pickle at a delicatessen near college for lunch, and another tinned-meat savoury in the evening, with vegetables, cheese and biscuits, or a piece of fruit. For a while after Christmas, there was also some chocolate.

The chocolate phase lasted from the time someone sent me a huge bar of it for Christmas until the time I realized I'd started to get more headaches since I'd been having a square of it every day, so I made myself stop. I felt rather irritable for a while afterwards, but the feeling eventually passed off. I think I may have half-realized I'd become hooked on the stuff, but since I still had no concept of food addiction, I wasn't able to elaborate this insight.

When I emigrated to London to begin my PhD, the pattern of my life underwent a radical change. After a month in an overseas student hostel, where I had the cooked breakfast provided but prepared my evening meal from tins and bits in my room, I moved into the first of a series of bedsits with use of kitchen, a mode of existence I was to continue for the next eleven years. At this time I discovered two new constraints upon my diet: a more extreme degree of impecuniousness than I had ever experienced before and the necessity of preparing my meals rapidly so that I wouldn't be in the way in the kitchen at mealtimes. Both circumstances favoured the evolution of a less nutritious diet than I had been used to. My limited budget increasingly dictated the choice of the cheaper carbohydrates, supplemented by eggs and cheese, in preference to the costlier animal proteins. Fortunately, I lived near a good street market, so at least I managed to get enough fruit and vegetables.

Shortly after taking up residence in the first bedsit, I made one of the most stupid mistakes of my life: I switched from a substantial, cooked, meat-based breakfast to a quick roll with jam and marge and maybe a piece of fruit with my coffee. This regimen meant that I could be out of the kitchen in the morning in next to no time. But it had major repercussions the rest of the day. By mid-morning I would find myself feeling weak, chilly, ravenous and unable to concentrate. Then I would either join my similarly-disposed colleagues for a quick cup of coffee and a biscuit in our common room or, if I was working in the library, which occupied the same building as the canteen, nip in for a coffee and a sausage roll, which just about kept me ticking over till lunchtime. After a light lunch in the canteen — soup, cheese and biscuits, and an apple — I would have a recurrence of the mid-morning crisis mid-afternoon and would again join my colleagues for tea and biscuits. It was only in the evening, after I'd had a more substantial meal, that I would start to feel recognizably human. But sometimes after supper I'd just suddenly fall asleep.

I was, of course, beginning to suffer from reactive hypoglycaemia on top of my by now multiple food addictions, without, of course, recognizing either of these two afflictions for what they were. Because so many of the people around me seemed to be having similar experiences — it was always the same crowd in the tearoom day after day and students in the classes I taught during the pre-break hour would also start to get peckish halfway through and rush out for sustenance the minute the class was over — I didn't realize that any abnormality was involved. Mid-morning and mid-afternoon ravenousness and inability to concentrate, relieved by inputs of coffee and tea, wheat, sugar and milk seemed to be the norm. Though it was staring me in the face, I didn't see the connection between the emergence of this syndrome and the change in my breakfast habits.

Thus when, after a year or so in the department, my mental health deteriorated to the point where I required treatment with anti-depressants, I failed to suspect the contribution that my diet was making to the general health rot that had set in. My circumstances at work were sufficiently unpleasant to appear to account quite adequately for my depressed state and none of the doctors I saw about it ever mentioned diet as a possible contributing factor in depression.

From that point onwards, my diet-related problems began to multiply. My jeans eventually brought to my attention the unwelcome fact that I had put on weight. A friend recommended an all-protein crash diet, which I tried for a fortnight. For the first few days I felt rotten, headachey and as if I were coming down with 'flu, but thereafter, as the weight dropped off at the rate of a pound a day with no hunger or irritability, I felt unusually well. After I reached my original weight, I was careful to avoid sugar, chocolate and most forms of starch and managed to keep my weight down. Of course, the significance of the initial withdrawal reaction escaped me.

Next, I lost whatever tolerance for alcohol I had ever possessed, which hadn't been much to begin with. I discovered the hard way fairly early on that alcohol and I didn't get on too well and after one disastrous encounter with a bottle of rum I became a very modest and reluctant social drinker. At parties I would accept a glass, take a few conspicuous sips, and then either leave the rest amongst the empty glasses or dispose of the contents when no one was looking – I would pour it into the flowerpots and hope the plants were thirsty. But at one party there were no plants, so I slipped my drink to the host's collie, who lapped it up and acted like a puppy until he fell asleep under the piano, whuffling and chasing dream rabbits.

With alcohol, I didn't like either the taste or the unpredictable results it seemed to have on me. Sometimes I would vomit, sometimes pass out, sometimes get a bit giggly, and sometimes fall asleep. I never drank enough to get depressed, but however little I drank, I invariably got at least a headache and a few times even a full-scale hangover. All in all, drinking just didn't seem worth it, but with all my food problems I hated to call extra attention to myself by not joining in.

What finally finished my career as a drinker was an evening spent with friends in Hampstead. They served sherry beforehand, wine with the meal, and brandy afterwards. Next thing I knew, I was lying on a bed with a blanket over me and a large and furiously purring tabby-cat digging herself a nest between my shoulder blades. In the morning, my hostess told me that I had fallen out of my chair after one sip of the brandy and they'd been unable to revive me in time to catch the last tube. That was the last time I accepted a drink. Enough was enough.

The next chapter in my food problems started with a visit to a neurologist when I started getting three sick headaches a week. He identified my longstanding condition as migraine, prescribed Cafergot, and advised me to try cutting out all the foods I suspected for a month and see what happened to the headaches. So out went meat (because of the fat), processed meats, tinned savouries, hard cheese, citrus, chocolate and eggs. The headaches tailed off. When I tested the suspects, all the meats – processed, fresh and tinned – gave me bad reactions, so I became more or less vegetarian for the next eight years. I occasionally ate fish and poultry, but avoided meat like the veritable plague. I still got an occasional migraine, but the new headaches came much less frequently and when they did occur were less violent and debilitating. Being vegetarian was a small price to pay – or so I thought.

The outcome of my vegetarian period was a host of health problems collectively much worse than the headaches. I became anaemic; the reactive hypoglycaemia worsened considerably; and I developed coeliac disease or something very much like it. Over and above these relatively well-defined complaints, I experienced a more or less definitive breakdown in my food tolerance. I expect that the high-cereal, high-milk, high-egg diet I adopted during this time was a factor in perpetuating the depression which went on almost constantly thoughout. Finally, I also developed hypothyroidism, but I don't know whether my diet contributed to this.

The one saving grace of this collapse of my health was that it occurred at a time when information about food-related problems was becoming more widely available to the public. It was also fortunate for me that the rot set in when I was old enough to question medical omniscience and to do something myself instead of continuing to suffer in silent acceptance of the many useless functional psychiatric labels — 'transient situational adjustment reaction', 'too introspective', 'anorexic', 'obsessional', 'hypochondriacal' and the like — that most of the doctors I saw used to dismiss my symptoms when preliminary biochemical investigations proved inconclusive.

Retreating to my own resources when medical help appeared bent on doing more harm than good, I read Mackarness's *Not All in the Mind*[1] and from there read on through the literature of food-related problems, food allergy, reactive hypoglycaemia, and coeliac disease in particular. As I began to understand more about the effects certain foods were having on me, I made, one by one, some major changes in my diet. To control the hypoglycaemia, I reduced my intake of carbohydrate to about 30g per day and found that as long as I maintained the restriction, the episodes of chill and drowsiness that overtook me after meals were largely eliminated. The mid-morning and mid-afternoon ravenousness and irritability largely disappeared and I felt a bit more energetic, despite my other continuing difficulties. Next, complete elimination of gluten stopped the malabsorption, and therapeutic doses of vitamins reversed the many deficiency sumptoms I had developed as a result. Finally, I tackled my remaining food allergies and intolerances, which meant the elimination of a lot of other foods – tomatoes, lettuce, corn, rice, green and red peppers, chemical additives, eggs, soya, cheese and all other milk products. I tested a lot of foods I hadn't been in the habit of eating — strawberries, peaches, potatoes, buckwheat, rhubarb, gooseberries, millet — and found that they didn't like me much either. At this point I had to resume eating meat, since there weren't many other forms of protein left. I expected a return of the headaches, but found that as long as I trimmed the fat off and didn't fry anything, I just about got by.

But my troubles were by no means over. In doing my reading I hadn't appreciated the importance of rotating foods, and before long I found myself unable to tolerate chicken, pork, tinned fish in oil, tinned shellfish, and liver. Eventually the light dawned and since then I have minimized further problems of intolerance by trying to rotate the foods I do eat as well as avoiding the ones that disagree with me the first time round.

Another problem, to which I have singularly failed to find a satisfactory solution, was surviving contact with hospitals without being made ill. My experience as an endocrine patient in search of a diagnosis seems to exemplify the problems that many allergic people encounter in their commerce with the health service. I must be one of the only people around who has had an adverse reaction to homoeopathic remedies, which are meant to be perfectly harmless. The consultant homoeopath I saw prescribed medicine which was dissolved in alcohol. He also prescribed some useless tablets, which, he told me when I wrote to him to find out what was in them, 'contained only lactose'. He added that he didn't think the medication 'could possibly have contributed' to my reaction. I reckoned that this disbelief revealed a certain lack of imagination – my GP had mentioned in his letter that I had food problems, but the consultant hadn't bothered to enquire about what these might be. Meanwhile, as soon as I started taking the medication, I began to get very bloated, headachey, and felt generally ill. After the alcohol, I went a bit crazy. I felt that the buildings were leaning over and about to collapse, that the clouds were racing unusually fast across the sky, and that these changes — which I recognized as subjective — were nonetheless fraught with special, if mysterious, personal significance. Colours were sharper and space distorted. I had to walk gently on the pavement to keep the surroundings, which seemed to have turned to glass, from crashing down in a million bits. I got some tablets from my GP the next day and the reaction passed off. it was extremely unpleasant and unnerving.

In another case, I had to withdraw from further investigations because the consultant wanted me to come into hospital for them. I felt this was out of the question because it would be practically impossible to avoid becoming ill through eating hospital food. Finally, I also withdrew from further ministrations by the third consultant I saw because she seemed unable or unwilling to appreciate the adverse effects that her investigations were having on me.

This experience is worth recounting in more detail because, despite the fact that the condition I was seeking help for was an orthodox, organic disorder rather than a symptom of my food problems, it seems to typify the predicament of the allergic person in medical situations. After correctly diagnosing my hypothyroidism on clinical grounds, this consultant sent me for an enormous battery of investigations, including, for some reason best known to her, a cholecystogram. The instructions for preparation mentioned a 'fatty meal' that would have to be consumed at one point in the procedure. I asked several nurses what this meant and was told that the radiographers would explain it to me at the time. I tried to explain why I needed to know, but it was no use. I was worried about what this 'fatty meal' might contain and didn't want to have an acute reaction whilst on the premises, where, if I passed out, I might find the situation taken out of my hands.

When the time came, I was handed a milky-looking coffee drink with no explanation. I said I had been told that they would tell me what was in it and said I wouldn't drink it until and unless I knew, since it could contain one of my allergens and make me very sick. The girl in white said she would try to find out and went off to confer with someone else. When she returned, she told me that the 'fat' part was egg yolk, but she'd been unable to find out about anything else in it. I said it would be better, then, if I didn't drink it, since egg was one of the things that disagreed with me. She replied that unless I drank it, the consultant would want the whole procedure repeated and that the X-rays I'd had so far would go to waste. Since the preparation had been pretty unpleasant — a stiff purge can be devastating to someone who has absolutely no need for it — I decided to take a chance. I needed treatment for my thyroid, which hadn't got better in the three years I had been seeking help for it, and going along with the consultant's requests seemed the only way I was ever going to get it.

I managed to keep the mixture down long enough to have the X-ray. Immediately it finished, I disappeared into the loo and vomited convulsively. I'd brought some safe food to break the fast, but after being so sick I felt too ill to eat it. I felt as though I were about to collapse and didn't want it to happen while I was still at the hospital — if they couldn't prevent reactions, they probably couldn't treat them properly either — so I got dressed and set out for home. On my way down the hill, I noticed that the colours looked particularly vivid and that the buildings seemed to be curving over. I leaned on a tree to steady myself. A little old lady trudging up the hill with a walking stick stopped to ask if I was all right. I wondered what she meant. It seemed a strange question to ask. Perhaps she was from the police? I nodded that I was all right. She looked doubtful, but continued up the hill. Maybe she thought I was drunk. I now felt I had to get home before I either collapsed or was apprehended, so I tottered off down the hill again, found the bus stop, and somehow managed to arrive at my flat. I found that if I touched the buildings as I walked by, the pavement seemed not to undulate beneath my feet. When I awoke after a few hours' sleep, I had a headache, felt ravenously hungry, chilled, weak and dopey. I recognized that my suspicions about the little old lady and about being apprehended were only part of the reaction. That afternoon I went to the surgery and got some more of the tablets I'd had after the homoeopathic reaction and they sorted me out within a day or so.

When I tried to tell the consultant about the adverse reaction, she seemed either unable or unwilling to appreciate that it had been precipitated by the mixture and apparently just decided I was crazy. Then she ordered a glucose tolerance test and insisted that I come into hospital to have it, so that I could fast under observation. I knew that there was absolutely no point in having the test because the medicinal glucose I would have to consume is derived from corn, one of my unsafe foods. I also knew that the observation that medicinal glucose can provoke nasty reactions in corn-sensitive people had been a part of the public record for many years.[2] But it is just not the patient's place to quote chapter and verse of the literature to a hospital consultant, especially not one who has already decided that the patient is crazy. The competence gap that is assumed to exist between knowledgeable doctors and ignorant patients is just too deeply entrenched a myth for it to be possible for someone in that situation to be able to argue, even if actually in possession of more authoritative knowledge. Thus when the consultant wrote to 'reassure' me that I needn't worry about the investigation 'because medicinal glucose is chemically pure and it doesn't matter if it is derived from corn or beet or wood', I didn't think it was worth bothering to send her a copy of the article. It wasn't my job to see to her postgraduate medical education. However, since by that time I was getting pretty desperate for some treatment for my thyroid, I decided to go along with the investigation, since complying seemed the only way I was ever going to get help. However, by insisting that I wouldn't come in unless I could bring my own safe food for breaking the fast and unless it could be kept under refrigeration until it was needed, I ensured — or so I thought — that glucose would be the worst allergen to which I was exposed.

I hadn't counted on the fact that at this particular teaching hospital they serve their glucose dissolved in orange squash which, of course, contains citrus and umpteen artificial additives. Taken on an empty stomach, this brew made me very sick indeed. Halfway through the test I vomited it up and collapsed on the bed. When I came to, the houseman told me that the consultant had wanted me to fast for much longer and now wanted me to get on with fasting so that the test could be repeated. Since I'd already had a fasting migraine the night before and since it was on the cards that the repeat test would have the same effect, if not worse, I told him I couldn't see the point. All I wanted was some thyroxine to make me better, not more unnecessary iatrogenic illness. He had no trouble understanding my point of view, lowered his voice, and said that he thought my best bet, then, was to find another consultant, since it seemed unlikely, the way things were going, that I'd get much real help from this one. He then asked me whether, as a personal favour, I'd be willing to sign myself out 'against medical advice', so it would look as though he'd advised me to stay and the consultant wouldn't vent her spleen on him. Since I had once worked for just such a consultant myself, I also had no trouble understanding his point of view, signed the pro forma, grabbed my case and disappeared, brimming with gratitude at this unexpected display of humanity.

That afternoon I saw my GP, so that he would have my version of what had happened before he got the consultant's. I told him I'd rather go on being ill under my own steam than with further 'help' from the specialist. He said it was up to me. Afterwards, I learnt that she had written to him to express 'concern about my mental state' and to assert that I was 'obsessional, hypochondriacal, and appeared anorectic'. Although one of my thyroid function tests had confirmed her clinical diagnosis of hypothyroidism, she was only prepared to offer me in-patient treatment for anorexia nervosa.

I didn't find out about this generous offer until some time after I had recovered from my thyroid condition on treatment with thyroid hormone, which I finally obtained on a private prescription from a medical friend. When I did find out what the consultant had in mind, I was truly appalled at the thought of what might have happened if the houseman hadn't warned me off in time. The standard treatment for anorexia nervosa these days consists of being put to bed, given drugs to increase appetite and reduce anxiety, and then fed double helpings of stodge, including all my worst allergens, at intervals throughout the day. How such a concerted metabolic assault could possibly have been intended to improve my hypothyroidism I simply cannot imagine. The experience left me very disillusioned with hospital medicine and I would now be reluctant to enter hospital except unconscious on a stretcher.

After I had stabilized on my dose of thyroxine — which my GP took over prescribing for me when it appeared obvious that it had been what I'd needed all along — I decided it would be prudent to get a Medic-Alert bracelet, so that if I *were* ever brought into hospital on a stretcher they'd be sure to continue to give it to me. Since more than one hidden health condition can be inscribed on the bracelet, I asked for it to include the information that I suffered from multiple food allergies, so that in addition to giving me thyroxine, they might be persuaded not to give me all the wrong things. I sent off the form, half expecting it to be returned with a curt note to the effect that this condition wasn't considered serious enough to warn doctors about, but the envelope that arrived in the post contained the bracelet, inscribed as I'd requested. I sincerely hope that I shall never have occasion to rely on it, but meanwhile I feel that bit safer going about each day. If the worst comes to the worst, the staff will have to believe I'm not just making up problems for the sake of being difficult.

At the present time, my propensity to adverse food reactions dominates my life more or less completely. Because I stick to my diet, I actually have very few symptoms to show for my affliction. But sticking to my diet is a full-time job in itself. There are so many foods I can't safely eat and some of the reactions can be so disabling, that I just don't take chances any more with food I haven't prepared myself or, at the very least, watched being prepared. I've found that with very few exceptions, it isn't safe to accept invitations to eat at friends' homes. If I eat socially at all, which I now do only vary rarely, it's *chez moi*, and often involves two lots of food, one for the guests and another for me. I avoid parties as a matter of principle most of the time and if I do attend, I forewarn my host or hostess that I won't be eating or drinking. Travelling is a nightmare and I only do so if I can bring enough safe food for the journey and do my own cooking at the other end. Residential events are out unless I can self-cater, which normally isn't possible. I've also had to turn down a number of invitations to speak out of town because there has seemed to be no way to get myself there and back in one piece. I have to assess all new possibilities in terms of whether they are likely to prove feasible from the point of view of safe eating; if they don't, they are automatically ruled out. I miss out on a lot this way.

Another consequence of the condition is that because I am dependent upon preparing my own food, I find I have to plan everything connected with eating a lot more closely than most people. Shopping has to be done most carefully, so that I can keep up some rotation of my proteins. Trips out of the house need to be worked out strategically, so that I'm not caught miles from home at a mealtime with nothing to eat. If I'm going to be out for any length of time, I've got to bring food with me. But I can't bring food for more than about two meals, because it tends to go off without refrigeration. So the radius within which most of my activity takes place has shrunk over the years. A friend once angrily called me a 'social cripple'. The term was cruel but not entirely inaccurate.

Another consequence is that, although I have my reactions under reasonable control most of the time, I still occasionally do get episodes of headache, tingling, general malaise, sudden drowsiness – amounting to narcolepsy – after meals, followed by bloating, mental dullness and more general malaise, which may last up to four or five days. These episodes occur after testing new foods which prove to be unsafe or deleted foods which haven't become safe yet. Because of these episodes, I tend to lose a considerable amount of time from productive work. Although I normally go into the office regardless of how I'm feeling, on such days I go about like a zombie and am not much use to anyone. In the evenings I get nothing useful done. If I don't just go to bed when I come in, the most I may accomplish for the whole evening is taking the rubbish out or watering the plants. Sometimes the symptoms may take a more benign form — a while ago I discovered that bananas now make me come out in a rash — but most of my reactions are of the incapacitating variety.

As a result of my condition, I have also found that my personality, such as it is, has been distorted in a number of ways. My three years of traipsing around the health service in search of some thyroxine have given me what would amount to a phobia of hospitals and of seeing doctors, if it weren't entirely rational and adaptive. The thought of ingesting gluten has the same effect on me. I tested it once and got a full-scale return of malabsorption, a long-drawn-out low-grade headache accompanied by feelings of impending doom, and a spate of paranoid ideas. The reaction was quite similar to the two iatrogenic reactions I described earlier, except that they didn't include a return of malabsorption. The thought that I might get such a devastating reaction again — all I'd done was test one biscuit — is enough to keep me on the straight and narrow, and curtails any tendency I might have had towards adventurousness. Moreover, the need for all the minute scrutiny of the details on the ingredients and eating arrangements leads to a certain degree of obsessiveness which goes completely against my nature. I'm not normally the overconscientious type; I can take most things as they come. But with food, all the fine print has to be worked out in advance and if for any reason it isn't or can't be, I get very uptight. I have often tried to explain to people who seemed bent on misunderstanding my concern that I'm not worried about detail for detail's sake, but because getting the details right is the only way to make sure I'm not going to become suddenly, and possibly violently, ill. Some people seem able to appreciate the distinction, but not all of them seem willing to try. Being treated as if I were pathological on the basis of behaviour aimed solely at preventing pathology irritates me enormously. It's bad enough to feel like a freak without having to put up with being treated like one.

The only good thing about my condition, that I can think of, is that it has enabled me to apply a more than academic knowledge to help other people who have similar problems. It may also be that in the long run the rather retiring and regular lifestyle I've had to adopt, and the avoidance of many foods that are associated with the development of degenerative diseases of affluence will prove to be to my advantage, too. But generally speaking the condition — or conditions — have been a lifelong handicap on practically all fronts and a source of considerable distress.

2.

A Group of People

'One man's meat is another man's poison'
Benjamin C, schoolboy, aged nine; Mrs Edna J, retired teacher, in her seventies; Alan B, freelance writer, mid-thirties; Dr Mike P, medical researcher, late-twenties; Jenny M, lecturer, mid-twenties; Mrs Margaret L, housewife and mother of four, mid-thirties; what do all these people have in common? Like Jack Spratt and his wife in the familiar nursery rhyme, they all share the common misfortune of reacting with symptoms when exposed to common foods and other substances that other people can tolerate without becoming ill.

Young Ben, who lives with his parents in a North London suburb, sticks to a careful rotation diet that his mother worked out for him with the help of a clinical ecologist and which keeps him on the rails. Ben comes from an allergic family and has had problems with allergies since infancy. As a small baby, eggs made him vomit. Iron tablets gave him eczema. Strawberries bring him out in a rash. Pork and bacon make his urine cloudy. Citrus, tomatoes and onions give him a sore anus. Milk and milk products, white flour, sugar, chocolate, cereal grains, artifical food colours, flavouring agents and preservatives make him hyperactive, unable to concentrate, with cloudy urine, urgency of micturition, swollen glands and catarrh. On top of his difficulties with foods, Ben also appears to be be allergic to wool, atropine eye drops, sun-tan creams, bubble bath, sticking plaster, vaccinations. As a baby, knitted nylon and certain brands of baby products disagreed with him. Twice when he has had EEGs, he has developed psoriasis of the scalp at the site where the electrode paste was applied.

People who do not understand Ben's difficulties regard him as 'badly behaved' and 'naughty'. Because of his diet, he misses out on some of his Cub Scout activities, has to come home for lunch or take his own meals, and he can't stay away from home without his mother to supervise the diet. If they go out for the day, all Ben's meals have to be brought along. His mother complains, too, how expensive it is to feed him — £2.50 per day when the questionnaire was filled in (1979) — and probably quite a lot more by now.

Ben's mother belongs to a self-help group for allergic people. She reports finding it a very great help, providing her with authoritative information, news of other parents' experiences, and support for her efforts to help her son. Since he has been on the diet, his teacher has noticed an improvement in his classroom behaviour and has co-operated by informing his mother when he has 'bad days' at school so that she can see whether they are related to dietary factors. Other people, however, are sceptical, she reports.

Although Ben takes quite a few nutritional supplements — calcium, vitamin B_6, zinc, and ascorbic acid — and sometimes a homoeopathic remedy if an adverse food reaction is suspected, it appears that he is still tending to become reactive to a wider range of substances. It remains to be seen whether his regimen will help him to avoid becoming allergic to everything as he gets older.

Mrs J, who lives in Sussex, used to suffer from migraine, giddiness, nausea, sore and puffy eyes, a crawling sensation of the skin, bouts of heart-thumping, smelly wind, sudden small bloodbursts in fingers or – occasionally – eyes, mouth ulcers, excessive tartar on the teeth, excessive tendency to bruising, an over-frequent need to pass water, and nettlerash. Her difficulties had been with her 'as long as she could remember'. She came from an allergic family. Her mother had migraine and eczema and both her sisters also suffered from migraine. From the age of five she had migraine occasionally, often with visual disturbances. When she reached her fifties, her troubles got worse. By her later sixties, she described her condition as 'really awful — I was never well'. One possible factor in this worsening was a long history of taking Cortisone, from her mid-forties until her late sixties, when she successfully weaned herself off it.

When Mrs J's migraines became continuous, she looked for more effective help than the Cafergot she had been prescribed. Eight visits to a clinical ecologist taught her all she needed to know to manage the condition herself. Her system of management is a four-day rotation diet with foods except milk taken not more than once a day. Mrs J says that this diet would have been a severe handicap during her professional life and that even now, in the comparative freedom of retirement, it limits her activities, and her husband's to a significant extent. The couple can only go out for meals with close friends. On holiday they have to go somewhere with self-catering facilities. However, she reported that recently they tried an experimental weekend at a good hotel that had an extensive à la carte menu at all meals. Although her rotation 'went haywire', Mrs J described the weekend as a great success, but added that probably a weekend was long enough and couldn't be repeated too often.

Alan B, living in the Midlands, is a chemical victim. His family history of allergy is not clear-cut, but he describes his father as preferring to avoid meat and sneezing a lot. Alan himself also has a tendency to develop nausea from eating meat or dairy products in any quantity and he also suffers from hay fever. In addition, he develops a rash after being in contact with detergents. But his main problem is that since he was in his late teens, he has suffered from hypersensitivity to chemical food additives, artifical colouring and flavouring agents, anti-oxidants, preservatives and the like. Monosodium glutamate also seems to affect him particularly badly.

Until his first year at university, Alan's allergies could be described as relatively uncomplicated. Although he had a range of substances that made him ill, he was fully aware of the connection between his symptoms and their precipitants and was never in any doubt about what was going on when he experienced them. Before starting his degree course, Alan worked for a year for a chemical company. His job involved spraying experimental pesticides that were being developed onto test crops and cleaning the warehouse in which the sprays were stored. The following year, out of the blue, he developed episodes of extreme anxiety, tension, confusion, giddiness, weakness and malaise, which seemed mainly to come on at mealtimes. When they occurred, these episodes could be incapacitating.

For the next twelve years Alan was, wrongly, thought to be mentally ill. He was given the full range of out-patient psychiatric treatments — drugs and more drugs, including some of the major tranquillizers, psychotherapy, behaviour therapy and counselling, all with no effect on these intermittent and disabling episodes. Despite this baffling affliction, he managed to obtain a postgraduate education, but then lost a number of jobs because his episodes were not understood. He was dismissed, in his own words, as 'a hopeless nutcase'. Eventually, however, he came to the attention of a clinical psychologist who realized that Alan wasn't 'neurotic' and encouraged him to keep a diet diary. In a few weeks of recording, he was able to identify his culprits. Now as long as he avoids packet foods with additives, Alan is able to pursue his new career as a freelance writer, but he is occasionally troubled by adverse reactions to petrol exhaust fumes and aerosol sprays, another legacy of his occupational sensitization to chemicals.[1]

Mike P, a medical researcher in his late twenties, works at a Scottish teaching hospital. Mike suffers from an isolated fixed allergy to green and red peppers. Exposure to even a small amount of pepper can cause prostration, violent diarrhoea and extreme dehydration. Mike seems to have inherited this condition from his mother, who also suffers from pepper allergy. Like his mother, he also gets migraines from time to time. Since he is medically qualified and since the precipitant of his dysentery-like symptoms is readily obvious, Mike has not needed to seek medical help with diagnosis. But on several occasions he has required emergency hospital treatment for his reaction to hidden peppers and once he nearly died. His condition makes him vulnerable to the inconsiderateness of others: on two occasions people have fed him peppers without telling him, 'to see what happened', even though he had warned them that the symptoms he got were particularly nasty. Needless to say, he was very angry and they were terribly embarrassed. Mike deals with his problem by avoiding peppers and by telling anyone who needs to know about his hypersensitivity. With the possibility of life-threatening reactions hanging over him, he quite understandably doesn't want to take unnecessary chances.

Jenny M, a science lecturer at a provincial university,

developed hypersensitivity to caffeine in coffee, tea and cola when she herself started at university and began to increase her consumption of caffeinated drinks. She would find herself sweating, her heart racing and palpitating, headachey, anxious, hot then cold, and would have to urinate more often than usual. Jenny's affliction appears to be fairly isolated: she doesn't know of any family history of allergy and also has no other forms of environmental intolerance. After having many problems with these episodes, she saw a GP who recognized the cause of her difficulties and told her to cut out caffeine, which she did. Over the intervening years, Jenny has managed to build up some degree of tolerance and can now manage one cup of coffee a day without ill effects. Although by contrast to some of the other respondents in the study Jenny is relatively lightly afflicted, she still finds her condition a problem at times. She reports that some of her friends think it 'rather strange' that she is unable to drink as they do. At college, when people invited her for coffee, they rarely had anything else available. Now she finds it 'a rather antisocial problem' and it is all the more annoying because she is very fond of tea and coffee. She says the problem doesn't really stop her doing anything socially, but she finds it does rather spoil things like going out to dinner when everyone else finishes up with coffee and she can't.

In the past, Jenny used to find it very hard to say 'no' if someone she didn't know very well, as a favour, made her a cup of tea or coffee without asking her first. Not wanting to offend them, she'd drink it and often would make herself ill in this way. Now she finds that saying 'no' isn't as much of a problem. She's older and more confident and also finds that many people tend to be more understanding about other people's dietary peculiarities. More often, too, they'll have an alternative to coffee and tea available to serve to guests who don't drink them.

Margaret L, living in Devon with her husband and four young children, has fixed allergies to a number of foods including onion, the mere smell of which can make her feel nauseous. Sometimes she also vomits. She reported that once when she was in hospital she ate a tomato that had been next to an onion and brought that up too. The smells of meat and fish can also affect her. She also gets a dry throat from smelling other people's cigarette smoke. The family are all non-smokers; her eldest child, Peter, has this reaction too. Although Margaret's own family history of allergy is not very strong (an aunt suffered from migraine) all four of her children – Peter, ten; Howard, eight; Hilary, six; and Corinne, four – have allergies. At four weeks of age, Corinne had diarrhoea from a certain brand of baby milk, resulting in sixteen dirty nappies per day, even though the milk was greatly diluted. Peter appears to be hypersensitive to sweets: after eating one, his ear swells up and becomes hot and red; the reaction can last an hour. After eating a few plain peanuts, both Peter and Howard have been sick and had diarrhoea, and Howard also developed difficulty in breathing. They were both ill enough to stay off school the rest of the day. Hilary reacts badly to soya beans. Howard became uncontrollable after eating grapes and Corinne is 'twice as hyperactive as usual' after eating a particular brand of dried raisins.

In order to help her allergic family, Margaret feeds them only pure, unadulterated foods. She makes her own bread and her own homemade sweets for the children. She gives them goat's milk, which they seem better able to tolerate than cow's milk. When they go to parties or are otherwise out for the day, she sends food along for them.

Margaret doesn't appear to have had much help from orthodox medicine. She says her allergic difficulties seemed to start in childhood after she had a bad reaction to penicillin and developed erythema nodosum, but her reactions to onion, fish and meat were not so severe when she was a child. In her teens, she developed abdominal difficulties and was sent to specialists for investigations, but they proved to be unable to help her. In her late teens, her parents finally took her to a naturopath, who suggested that she become 100 per cent vegetarian, which she did. Her difficulties lessened. Thereafter, she had a prolonged reaction to pethidine, which she was given during Peter's birth.

By contrast, in dealing with her children's allergic difficulties, Margaret has had help from a number of groups for sufferers — Sanity, and the Hyperactive Children's Support Group in particular. Through Sanity she obtained some helpful blood tests for herself and all the children. The tests confirmed many of the observations she had made by herself. The Hyperactive Children's Support Group list of 'banned foods' has been helpful in identifying culprits. Her history of adverse drug reactions has made her chary of exposing the children, so she has attended a homoeopathic clinic instead; she finds that their remedies do not cause bad reactions either for her or her offspring. Only in extreme circumstances will she use an orthodox drug such as Piriton. Her view is that it is better to prevent symptoms occurring in the first place than to pay for unconcern with illness.

These six people illustrate some of the diversity in the population of allergic people. How many are there who share these problems? And do they have any common denominators besides their tendency to react with symptoms to environmental factors that leave their unaffected fellows untouched? At the present time, hard and fast answers to these important questions are difficult to come by.

Immunology textbooks seem to agree that approximately ten per cent of the population suffer from so-called atopic or Type I allergy (e.g. eczema, hay fever, asthma, allergic rhinitis). At the opposite extreme, Dr Richard Mackarness, Britain's leading proponent of clinical ecology, has estimated that thirty per cent of people attending GPs have symptoms traceable exclusively to food and chemical problems and that an additional thirty per cent have symptoms partially traceable to these causes.[2] While we have at present no way of estimating the prevalence of these sorts of problems in people who do not attend GPs, it seems reasonable to think that a proportion of non-attenders is probably also affected. A conservative estimate, then, might place the prevalence rate at perhaps around fifty per cent of the population, but if all forms of hypersensitivity to environmental substances are included, the rate might probably come closer to between eighty and ninety per cent, since many people who attend their GPs have symptoms other than the ones they consult him about and many people with mild and transient symptoms, such as, perhaps, a rash from sticking plaster or an upset stomach after a fast-food snack, do not bother to consult their GPs.

With such a high proportion of the population likely to be affected by such a heterogeneous group of afflictions, it might be more useful to ask what kinds of people do *not* become intolerant of environmental factors! To answer this question, however, also remains a task for the future, when epidemiological studies have been conducted and a population of hardy individuals who are able to withstand the ecological assaults that the rest of us succumb to has been isolated. Meanwhile, these considerations lead to the conclusion that individuals who develop ecological hypersensitivity are most probably too diverse to make it worth while to seek common denominators of the sociological variety. Biological and ecological factors, such as an hereditary predisposition to allergy and a history of bottle feeding in infancy, dietary deficiencies, particularly of essential fatty acids and the mineral and vitamin co-factors required for their conversion to hormones called prostaglandins, necessary for the efficient functioning of the immune system, and also a history of exposure to sensitizing chemicals are likely to explain more of the variation between sufferers and non-sufferers than superficial demographic characteristics. Of these, only the first, the question of family history, can receive even a partial answer from the results of the survey.

When the survey was originally planned, I had hoped to find fifty people, equal numbers of either sex, from as wide a range of backgrounds as possible. The final sample turned out to be much larger — eighty five people — but contained roughly three times as many women as men. These people came from all over the country and were drawn from a variety of sources. The story of how they came to take part in this research is worth telling here because it sheds some light on the situation of allergic people in Britain today.

Because the people I work with know of my interest in allergy, many of them have spoken to me about their special problems in this department. When the questionnaires for the study came back from the Rehabilitation Unit where the stencils had been run off, I posted a notice on the bulletin board asking for allergic volunteers to fill it in. Over the next several months I had many enquiries about the study and quite a few people volunteering to fill in the questionnaires themselves or to get a friend or relative with allergies to fill one in. Several people commented that this was the first time anyone had shown interest in what it was like to live with their sorts of problems and wanted to take the opportunity to make their views known.

Then I wrote to the Secretary of the McCarrison Society, who at the time was Dr Barbara Latto, to ask whether a request for participants could appear in the Society's Newsletter, which circulates to many food-conscious people all over the country. As a result of this appeal, I heard from several private individuals in distant parts of the country and also from three important organizations for sufferers. Mrs Amelia Nathan Hill rang to ask if I would like her to distribute copies of the survey questionnaire to members of her Action Against Allergy, which she told me at the time had a national membership of several thousand people. Then Dr Richard Mackarness of Park Prewett Hospital in Basingstoke wrote to ask about handing out copies to members of his Chemical Victims Club for his former patients. Finally, I also heard from Mrs Sally Bunday, Honorary Secretary of the Hyperactive Children's Support Group, offering to send some copies to mothers of hyperactive children who were following special diets for the control of their condition. I gratefully accepted all offers, reserved a drawer of my filing cabinet for the returned questionnaires, and by the end of 1980 had collected a total of eighty five.

The willingness of three leading self-help groups to put their resources at the disposal of an unknown investigator and the deluge of questionnaires that followed — many of which were accompanied by letters, copies of allergy test results, and other documentation — points to a great keenness amongst sufferers everywhere to make their special difficulties known. Both the great diversity amongst participants and the great variety in the problems they described emphasize the wide-ranging effects that allergy can have upon its victims. And the high degree of similarity in many people's problems that shines through all the differences points to the existence of a common core of need for better public understanding and better medical and food supply services in the community. From here onwards, the story belongs to the eighty five respondents.

Demographic Characteristics of the Group

Though the survey questionnaire (a copy of which is given in Appendix A) was to be completed anonymously, respondents were asked to indicate their age, sex and occupation.

Table 1:Ages of survey respondents

Age range	M	F	All
0—9	4	0	4
10—19	3	5	8
20—29	6	13	19
30—39	1	12	13
40—49	2	16	18
50—59	3	12	15
60—69	1	6	7
70—79	0	1	1

The final sample contained twenty males with a mean age of 28.6 years (S.D. 18.89) and sixty five females with a mean age of 40.48 years (S.D. 14.85). The age range for the group as a whole was 2–70 years and respondents were well distributed across decades, as shown in Table 1. The table shows that all but two groups — girls under ten and men over seventy — were represented in the survey sample.

The social-class composition of the group was not easy to describe, because a large proportion of respondents (thirty two of eight five or 37.65 per cent) fell into uncodable categories: one was a pre-school infant, nine were school children, three students, two retired, sixteen housewives and one self-employed; in these cases no indication of the occupation of head of household or the actual nature of the respondent's own occupation was given. Therefore the analysis has had to be confined to the remaining fifty three respondents who indicated a codable occupation. These findings are shown in Table 2.

Table 2: Social class composition of survey group

Social class	M n = 20		F n = 65		All n = 85	
	n	%	n	%	n	%
I	5	25.00	11	16.92	16	18.82
II	4	20.00	20	30.77	24	28.24
III	2	10.00	9	13.85	11	12.94
IV	—		—		—	
V	—		—		—	
Unclassified	9	45.00	25	38.46	34	40.00

The sample included medical practitioners, university lecturers, clinical psychologists, nurses, teachers, typists, office-machine operators, a computer-systems analyst, a school inspector, a sheet-metal worker, a chartered civil engineer, a hospital administrator, a retailer, salesmen, a department-store buyer, freelance writers, accountants, clerical workers, a telegraphist, a political agent, a licensee, a hotelier and a librarian.[3]

The predominantly middle-class composition of the group is a direct result of the way the sample was recruited; middle-class people are more likely than others to avail themselves of the help of self-help groups. But we cannot conclude that they are any more likely than others to suffer allergies.

Table 3: Geographical Distribution of survey sample

Region	f	%
Home counties	21	24.71
London	19	22.35
South-east	16	18.82
South-west	5	5.88
Scotland	5	5.88
North	5	5.88
Midlands	4	4.71
West	4	4.71
Not stated	6	7.06

Geographical Distribution

Seventy nine of the eighty five respondents indicated an address. The counties were analysed according to broad regional groupings and the frequencies of residence in each were established. These results are shown in Table 3.

The residential pattern of the survey-group members reflects both the location of the self-help groups involved and also the fact that a proportion of respondents was personally contacted by the London-based investigator. Although the sample has a strong South-Eastern bias, however, members were found in the other major regions of the country.

Family History

Respondents were asked whether they knew of any family history of disorders similar to or related to their own. The results of this enquiry showed that some ninety per cent of all respondents came from allergic families. The true proportion may actually be higher, because in five cases respondents replied that they didn't know. The figures are given in Table 4.

Table 4: Family history of allergic disorder (including migraine) in survey respondents

	M n = 20		F n = 65		All n = 85	
	n	%	n	%	n	%
No	0	0	3	4.62	3	3.53
Don't know	2	10	3	4.62	5	5.88
Yes	18	90	59	90.77	77	90.59

There appears to be no difference between the sexes in the

rate of positive family histories. The results suggest that most people with food and chemical hypersensitivity are likely to be endowed from birth with a potentially allergically reactive constitution, but we can't necessarily conclude that most people who have inherited an allergic tendency will necessarily have problems with foods and chemicals.

While many respondents gave details of their family backgrounds of allergic problems, in other cases the information given was not very detailed; thus it was not possible to assess the degree of specificity of the constitutional tendency, as Gerrard and his co-workers have done.[4] These investigators found that there was a strong association between certain allergic disorders, such as asthma, hay fever, recurrent rhinitis, recurrent bronchitis, and eczema, but not urticaria, in parents and their offspring. In future it would be interesting to determine whether food and chemical problems in one or both parents are also likely to appear in offspring. But to answer this question, a different method of study would be required.

Past Personal History

For most of the respondents of both sexes, environmental hypersensitivity was not only constitutional but also lifelong. In answer to the question about the history of their own personal difficulties, the majority reported onsets of difficulties occurring before they reached adulthood. These results are shown in Table 5.

Table 5: Pre-adult vs. adult onsets in men and women

Time of onset	M n = 20		F n = 65	
	n	%	n	%
Before adulthood	16	80.00	47	72.30
In adulthood	10	50.00	60	92.30

The percentages add up to more than 100 per cent because many people reported more than one onset. Although the difference between the rate of adult onsets falls short of statistical significance (x^2 = 0.63), there does seem to be a tendency for a higher proportion of women to report an onset in the adult years. However, we must not forget that the mean age of the female sample was considerably higher than that of the male sample, so that the higher rate of adult onsets in females may simply reflect the fact that the women had had, on average, more time during their adulthood in which to have onsets. But it may also be the case that the effect is a real one.

In trying to decide between these two explanations, we may consider the additional information which respondents gave about their onsets. They were asked how the condition had started; the breakdown of their replies is shown in Table 6.

Table 6: Time and circumstances of onsets

When difficulties started	M n = 20		F n = 65		All n = 85	
	n	%	n	%	n	%
Before adulthood						
Present since birth	9	45.00	6	9.23	15	17.65
Started in infancy	3	15.00	5	7.69	8	9.41
Started in childhood	2	10.00	21	32.31	23	27.06
Started in adolescence	2	10.00	15	23.08	17	20.00
In adulthood						
After stress	5	25.00	10	15.38	15	17.65
After pregnancy	—	—	7	10.77	7	8.24
Gradually	2	10.00	12	18.46	14	16.47
Out of the blue	2	10.00	15	23.08	17	20.00
Unspecified	1	5.00	11	16.92	12	11.12

While they are by no means definitive, these findings suggest that different factors may contribute to the appearance of allergic phenomena in members of the two sexes. The fact that roughly five times as many males as females reported difficulties present since birth and twice as many reported problems in infancy are consistent with the general finding that male infants and children tend to be more vulnerable than females to a variety of disorders.[5] The finding is unlikely to be due simply to the fact that many of the male respondents were young boys, whose mothers filled in the questionnaire on their behalf, since the mothers of the young girls in the sample did not report as many early difficulties with their daughters. The higher rate of onsets in females at adolescence suggests that hormonal factors also play a role in the manifestation of allergic tendencies and the importance of pregnancy as a precipitant adds weight to this suggestion. Stress also appears to be a factor for both men and women. The higher proportions of both gradual and sudden onsets in women may also point to the operation of hormonal factors, but environmental influences, such as differences in rate of exposure to anaesthetics, cosmetic chemicals, detergents and household cleansers, gas cookers, drugs and dangerous foods may also play a part.

The fact that many respondents reported more than one onset, occurring at different ages, emphasizes the lifelong nature of the problems which possession of an allergically reactive constitution may entail. While some childhood afflictions may show improvement in later life, others may persist and be joined by a host of new sensitivities. These possibilities were the topic of a separate enquiry.

Stability and Change in Allergic Problems

Respondents were asked whether their allergic difficulties had changed or remained the same since they had started.

Table 7: Changes in sensitivity

Category	M n = 20		F n = 65		All n = 85	
	n	%	n	%	n	%
Difficulties remained the same	8	40.00	23	35.38	31	36.47
DK, too early to tell	2	10.00	8	12.31	10	11.76
New sensitivities developed	0	0	9	13.85	9	10.59
Some decrease in sensitivities	3	15.00	12	18.46	15	17.65
Some increase in sensitivities	3	15.00	14	21.54	17	20.00
Condition fluctuates	2	10.00	3	4.62	5	5.88
Worse before getting better	2	10.00	7	10.77	9	10.59
Some control with treatment	9	45.00	38	58.46	47	55.29
Full control with treatment	1	10.00	6	9.23	7	8.24

Unfortunately, the majority of respondents apparently took the question to refer to their present difficulties; some, but not all, differentiated between their sensitivities *per se* and changes in symptomatic expression as a result of treatment, so that the results are less than clear cut. They are given in Table 7.

The table shows that nearly forty per cent of respondents reported that their conditions remained essentially unchanged once they had started. Over sixty per cent reported that they had achieved at least some degree of control over their condition with treatment which, in most cases – as we shall see in a later chapter – meant effective avoidance of offending substances. Roughly ten per cent were still too young for the question to be meaningful or had developed their symptoms too recently to be able to tell whether significant change would occur. The proportions reporting increase and decrease in sensitivity were approximately the same, around twenty per cent. Another fifteen per cent reported fluctuations in their condition from time to time, increase in sensitivity often being associated with a pile-up of other stresses. And ten per cent, all of them women, reported the development of new sensitivities since their present main condition had started. Most of these reports referred to an increase in the range of foods or chemicals causing difficulties rather than to change in the class of substances that precipitated symptoms.

These findings suggest that for a majority of sufferers the manifestations of their constitutional allergic tendency probably do not remain static. Some may experience improvement, in that either they cease to react at all or to react less severely to certain allergens; others may become more sensitive to the same allergens and/or develop sensitivities to new ones, often unpredictably and erratically. The instability of the condition, and particularly its liability to deteriorate, can be a source of much additional distress to some sufferers. As we shall see in later chapters, some allergic people may live in fear not only of developing symptoms when they are unable to avoid contact with their allergens but also of losing what tolerance of the environment they may still possess and then becoming, like ex-pop singer Sheila Rossall, 'allergic to the twentieth century'. Obviously not all sufferers are so severely affected, but for those who are showing signs of a deteriorating tolerance, the future can be frightening to contemplate.

This, then, is the group of people whose reports provide the basis for this book: people of all ages, from many walks of life, from all over the country — all have in common their tendency to develop symptoms upon exposure to one or more substances in the environment that other people appear to be able to tolerate with impunity.

Next we need to examine the substances that provoke their symptoms. This will be the topic of the next chapter.

3.

Allergens

The first question on the survey questionnaire read as follows:

Are there any foods, drinks, or chemical substances which are either swallowed or inhaled that you are aware of having unpleasant or unusual reactions to? If so, what are they and what are the reactions they provoke? (Please include anything you feel pretty sure about, even if the reaction only occured once.)

In this and the following chapter we will consider the group's answers to this question. In this chapter we will be concerned with the precipitants of their symptoms and in the next chapter with the symptoms themselves.

Although the question only asked specifically about foods and chemical ingestants and inhalants, the respondents did not hesitate to mention other sorts of substances that also cause them to experience symptoms.

Their replies to the question were subjected to content analysis using inductively derived categories that classified substances according to general type, e.g. foods, food additives, pollens, metals, natural and synthetic fabrics, and the like. In addition, a few special categories such as coffee and tea were included separately rather than being subsumed under the general heading of foods. The general sort of categorization was chosen in preference to a more exhaustive one in order to keep the analysis within manageable limits. At a later stage, a separate analysis of individual foods was also conducted.

A Note on Terminology

Since the material under analysis consists of self-report data, we have no way of being absolutely certain whether all the substances named as causing difficulties exert their noxious effects by orthodox immunological means. In fact, it seems virtually certain that not all of them could do: one respondent, for instance, was a sufferer from coeliac disease, a disorder characterized by malabsorption of the nutrients in foods because of damage to the absorptive surface of the villi in the small intestine, caused by intolerance of gluten, found in wheat, rye, barley and oats, but a disorder which is not an allergy in the usual limited sense. Another respondent suffered from lactose intolerance, a condition due not to allergy but to a deficiency in the enzyme lactase, which enables the milk sugar to be broken down properly in the body. A third respondent was hypersensitive to the pharmacological action of caffeine, a centrally-acting drug which has the potential to induce toxic reactions in anyone provided a sufficiently high dose is taken. Her problem was not allergy to coffee and tea but rather the possession of a lower threshold for caffeine toxicity than most people seem to possess — a quantitative rather than a qualitative difference from the norm. Similarly, the several young children whose hyperactive behaviour was aggravated by artificial food colours, flavours and preservatives, and who improved when these chemicals were removed from their diet may also be hypersensitive to their pharmacological effects rather than allergic to them. Why then, it seems fair to ask, are these people's dietary culprits called 'allergens' if they are not truly *allergic* to them?

The answer — which I fear probably won't satisfy many immunologists — is that these substances are called allergens for want of a better term. The English language lacks a technical, generic name for substances that cause symptoms in hypersensitive people without implying anything about mechanisms. In colloquial English, on the other hand, such substances are called allergens. Thus when Snoopy declares he is 'allergic to morning', people smile in recognition; it is perfectly clear to everyone what he means. So although the term 'allergens' may sometimes be used here in a sense that is not

100 per cent accurate technically, most readers are likely to have less difficulty in understanding what is meant than if some unfamiliar and inelegant neologism were used to designate the source of some people's difficulties.

In a book on the causes of allergy it would, of course, be misleading to use a single term for all substances that cause people to develop symptoms regardless of the mechanisms by which the symptoms are brought about. But in a book which is fundamentally concerned not with the causes but rather with the everyday effects of living in a body that reacts in uncommon ways to common substances, the terminological imprecision that will sometimes occur is less serious. The majority of what will be called allergens undoubtedly *are* allergens — and several respondents included copies of their allergy-test results to prove it. In any case, the main point of the enquiry is not to find out what people are allergic to, but to discover the ways in which their unusual sensitivities cause problems for them in their efforts to live normal lives in the community. From this point of view it is relatively unimportant whether someone is allergic to a substance, intolerant of it, lacks an enzyme necessary to deal with it, has a low threshold for its toxicity, or reacts adversely to it for some other reason — the problems of trying to avoid it and of dealing with symptoms when avoidance proves impossible are basically the same, and quite often the same substances are involved.

Bearing these conditions in mind, let us now proceed to look at the analysis of the results.

Number of Types of Allergen Reported

The range of the numbers of allergen types reported was approximately the same for both sexes: men reported between one and fourteen and women between one and thirteen. In terms of the average number reported by the two sexes, there was a slight tendency for women to be more extensively affected. Men reported an average of 3.15 (S.D. 2.97) types of allergen versus an average of 4.82 (S.D. 2.82) for women. It is clear that for both men and women, multiple sensitivities are the rule.

The numbers of allergen types reported by the group as a whole were plotted as a frequency histogram, as shown in Figure 1. The graph shows that the group tends to subdivide into three sorts of people: forty two individuals who reported

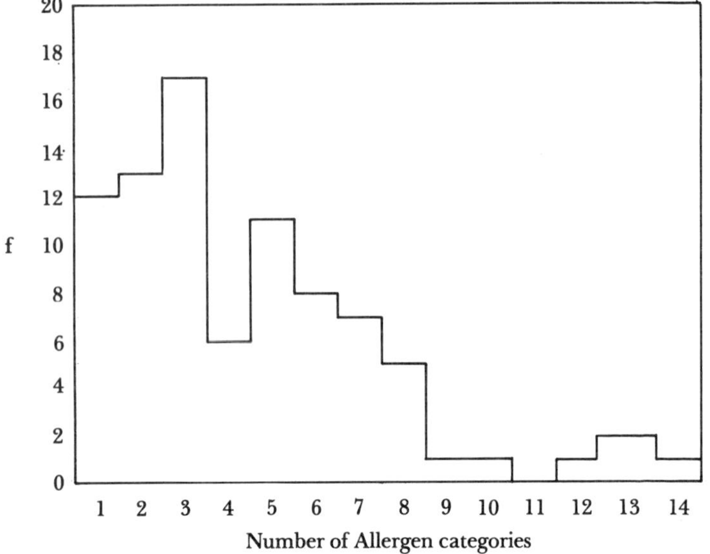

Figure 1.

between one and three types of allergen, thirty nine who reported between four and ten, and another four who reported between twelve and fourteen. Thus the group as a whole seems to be divided more or less equally between people who may be considered to be relatively mildly affected in terms of the range of types of substances to which they are hypersensitive (forty-two) and people who in the same terms may be regarded as more severely affected (forty-three). In the chapter on limitations arising from allergic conditions we will examine the question whether the range of sensitivities a person reports is related to the overall severity of the condition, in terms of the degree to which it limits participation in social life and the number of types of symptoms which it produces.

Individuals with Only One Type of Allergen
So far we have seen that multiple sensitivities are the rule, since only twelve of the eighty-five respondents reported reacting to only one type of allergen. An analysis of these twelve individuals reveals, further, that even amongst people who react adversely to only one category of substance, multiple sensitivities within that category also predominate. The

relevant information about these twelve respondents is shown in Table 8.

Table 8: The twelve individuals with only one category of allergen

MALES

No.	Age	Category	Specifics
1	25	Foods	shellfish, barley water, excess sugar and starch excess milk and cheese
2	29	Foods	red and green peppers
3	22	Gluten	wheat, rye, barley, oats
4	25	Detergents	washing powder
5	52	Foods	white bread, garlic, shellfish, fish
6	40	Foods	mushrooms, tomatoes, fruit seeds

FEMALES

No.	Age	Category	Specifics
7	46	Foods	flours, pork, milk, beef, runner beans, spinach, pears, strawberries
8	57	Foods	cooked cheese, chocolate
9	51	Foods	'all foods except oatmeal, potato, lamb, goat's milk'
10	35	Foods	wheat, wheat products, eggs
11	12	Foods	wheat, rye, barley, oats, peas, peanuts, runner beans, beet sugar, baked beans
12	52	Foods	milk and milk products, white flour and products, foods with large amounts of calcium

From the information in the table we can see that foods are by far the most common single category reported by the group members: eleven of the twelve mentioned them. Although equal numbers of males and females reported single categories, the condition seems to be more common in the males, since the male sample was considerably smaller. The figures represent thirty per cent of the men as against 9.23 per cent of the women who took part in the survey. There were two other women respondents with what might have been counted as single class susceptibilities if a different method of analysis had been used.

One lady reported an isolated hypersensitivity to egg, whether consumed or inhaled or touched (in the form of egg shampoo). But she was counted as reacting adversely to both foods and

Table 9: Frequency of types of allergen reported by the survey sample

Frequency	%	Category
82	96.47	Foods
32	37.65	Food additives and contaminants
29	34.12	Alcohol
		Coffee
26	30.59	Petrochemical fumes
21	24.71	Tea
19	22.35	Detergents, soaps and shampoos
17	20.00	Perfumes and cosmetics
11	12.94	Aerosol sprays
		Drugs
		Pollens and plants
10	11.76	Dust
8	9.41	Tobacco
		Moulds and yeast
7	8.24	Other chemicals
6	7.06	Animals, fur, hair, danders
5	5.88	Metals
		Synthetic fabrics
4	4.71	Gluten
		Antibiotics
		Water
		Natural fabrics
		Plastics
3	3.53	Anaesthetics
		Strong smells
		Sticking plasters
2	2.35	Dyes (contactants)
		Insects
		Travelling
1	1.18	Lactose
		Noise
		Cold
		Vaccines
		Pesticides

shampoos. The second reported hypersensitivity to caffeine in coffee and tea and was counted as reacting adversely to both substances, since each comprised a separate category in the analysis. But even if these two women had been included, the proportion of males with single types of sensitivity would still have been quite a bit higher.

It is clear from the table that if a person is allergic to something, the chances are very high that he or she will also be allergic to something else. The young man with an isolated hypersensitivity to washing powder is a minority of one within the entire survey sample.

The Allergens Themselves

The frequencies with which the allergen categories were mentioned are shown in Table 9. Since the sample was intended to consist of people with food and chemical problems, it is not surprising that substances in these two categories were most often named. The finding suggests that the method of recruiting subjects succeeded in its aim. Interestingly, the proportion of people who reported allergy to dust (11.76 per cent) and to pollens (12.94 per cent) is about the same as the ten per cent figures for the general population that are often quoted. While the findings do not tell us anything about the prevalence of food and chemical problems in the population at large, they do suggest that these sorts of difficulties are likely to be more common than the orthodox textbook-type allergies. At the very least, the results of this analysis show clearly that many people with food and chemical problems also react adversely to other types of allergens and that, conversely, at least some people with orthodox inhalant allergies will also react adversely to other types of substance, including foods and chemicals.

Particular Foods

The particular foods that respondents cited as causing them difficulties were analysed separately. The frequencies with which individual foods were mentioned are shown in Table 10.

Perhaps the most obvious fact that emerges from the table is that the foods that are part of the public stereotype of 'food allergy', that is, strawberries and shellfish, turn out to be relatively uncommon food allergens, being mentioned by only three and seven people respectively. By contrast, there is a very evident trend for the more common constituents of the average British diet — cereal grains, milk and dairy products, coffee and tea, alcohol, sugar, egg, chocolate, citrus, and food

Table 10: Foods mentioned as causing symptoms

Frequency	Food
52	Wheat and wheat products
34	Cows' milk
32	Food additives and contaminants
31	Cheese
29	Coffee, alcohol
28	Chocolate
24	Citrus
23	Corn
22	Egg, cane sugar
21	Oats, tea
18	Rye
17	Rice
16	Apple, banana
14	Barley
13	Fish
12	Butter, pork, tomato
11	Yoghurt, cream, onion
9	Chicken, peanut
8	Grape/raisin, brassicas, yeast
7	Ice-cream, beef, pork products, shellfish, potato
6	Beetroot/sugar, soya, confectionary, MSG, carrot, fruit drinks, honey
5	Millet, lamb, mushroom, pear, plum, currant, peach, nuts, runner beans, food combinations, instant foods
4	Gluten, smoked foods, lettuce, glucose, parsnip, broad beans, tinned foods, garlic
3	Buckwheat, turkey, animal fats, vegetable oils, strawberries, red and green peppers, jam, cake mixes
2	Margerine, corned beef, starch, shortbread, Melon, baked beans, cherries, 'beans', decaffeinated coffee, pineapple
1	Lactose, fruit seeds, peppercorns, coriander, mustard, curry, fructose, swede, butter beans, turnip, celery, cucumber, courgette, spinach, vinegar, barley water, protein-free flour, gluten-free flour, liver, foods with large amounts of calcium, cola, dried fruits, parsley, tapioca, gooseberry, apricot, radish, watercress, lentil, avocado, chicory, dried beans, coconut, Jerusalem artichoke, Bovril, Camp coffee, Marmite, Horlicks, Lucozade, Worcester sauce, Perrier water

additives — to be most often reported as causing people's symptoms. We will return to this point later on.

Comparative Findings

How reliable are these findings? It is a fair question, for if the findings were a purely random occurrence it would be hazardous to base any conclusions on them. One way of checking the reliability of frequency data such as these is to compare the frequencies found in two samples of subjects who were studied independently. While surveys of this nature that might be used for comparative purposes do not appear to have been done in Britain, some similar findings have been reported in the United States. In 1970, for example, Speer published a list of the incidence of food allergens in 1000 patients of all ages seen in his private allergy practice.[1] For Speer's group as a whole, allergies to the following were found most frequently. The figures in brackets refer to the numbers out of 1000 who were found to be allergic to the food:

milk	(679)	tomato	(133)
chocolate-cola	(400)	wheat	(118)
corn	(302)	apple	(75)
citrus	(272)	cinnamon	(71)
egg	(259)	rice	(65)
legumes	(229)	food colours	(64)

Of the top twelve allergenic foods, seven are the same in both lists. Rice, apple and tomato also figured high on the British list. Despite minor differences, there is clearly a general agreement between the present findings and Speer's; it seems safe, therefore, to conclude that the present findings are probably fairly representative.

Coffee and Tea

Because of contemporary interest in the noxious effects of coffee,[2] it seemed worthwhile to examine the degree of overlap between the twenty nine people who reported problems with coffee and the twenty one reporting difficulties with tea. This analysis showed that there were fifteen people who reported having problems with coffee but not tea, seven who mentioned problems with tea but not coffee, and fourteen who got symptoms from both. In the sample as a whole there were forty-nine people who reported problems with neither coffee nor tea. Though they are in the majority, it is worth considering that 42.35 per cent of the people in our sample had problems with coffee and/or tea. Given the number of social occasions in daily life where only coffee and tea are available to drink, we may begin to anticipate some of the social difficulties that allergic people are likely to encounter.

Cereal Grains and Milk

This combination of foods has received considerable public attention recently, not only because of the difficulties they cause for sufferers from coeliac disease and other conditions of gluten sensitivity,[3] but also because of recent findings concerning their probable role in the pathogenesis of schizophrenia.[4] When wheat and wheat products and milk and milk products were examined, it was found that seventeen of the eighty-five respondents reported difficulties with neither wheat nor milk, thirteen reported problems with milk but not wheat, nineteen mentioned problems with wheat but not milk, and thirty-six reported difficulties with both. When all cereal grains in addition to wheat were included in a separate analysis, the corresponding figures were: 16 (neither), 9 (milk only), 21 (grains only) and 39 (both). Thus nearly half the sample (45.88 per cent) reported getting symptoms from both cereal grains and grain products and milk and milk products while slightly under a fifth (18.82 per cent) had problems with neither. Fully four-fifths (81.18 per cent) of the sample were affected by one or other or both of these dietary staples. Coeliacs and schizophrenics are thus by no means the only people for whom these foods can be dangerous: most people who suffer from food allergy seem likely to have trouble with either or both of them.

Chemicals

With chemicals as with foods, people who are affected at all appear as a rule to have multiple sensitivities. People who reported adverse reactions to food additives mentioned an average of 1.84 types of additive as causing difficulties. Food colours were most frequently cited, being mentioned by twelve of the thirty two people who suffered from hypersensitivity to additives. Artificial flavours and preservatives were each mentioned by eleven respondents and another ten mentioned miscellaneous additives, additives generally, or products containing additives. Thus five mentioned instant, packet or convenience foods generally, four had difficulties with tinned foods because of residues from the lining, four mentioned artificially smoked foods, and six reported adverse reactions to monosodium glutamate (MSG).

With non-food chemicals, which were mentioned by a total of fifty-five people, the average number was three types of chemicals per person. Of the fifty-five, only seventeen mentioned difficulties with one type of chemical; the remaining thirty-eight had problems with at least two types and one had difficulties with as many as fourteen different types. The frequency counts of people mentioning particular types of chemicals have already been given in Table 9.

A separate analysis was done to see whether people who reported reacting adversely to food chemicals were also hypersensitive to non-food chemicals. There were nineteen respondents in the entire group of eighty five who reported no reactions to chemicals; eleven who reported reacting only to food chemicals; thirty four who reported reacting only to non-food chemicals; and twenty one who reacted to both food and non-food chemicals. A total of sixty-six respondents — or 77.65 per cent of the sample – reported reacting badly to at least one type of chemical. This means that people who are hypersensitive to foods would also seem to have a high probability of being hypersensitive to chemicals as well. Of course, it is also possible to react to chemicals but not to foods, as in the case of the young man with isolated hyperreactivity to washing powder, but the present findings suggest that this may be an uncommon state of affairs.

Some Implications of the Findings

We noted earlier that the most commonly reported food culprits tended to be amongst the most common constituents of the typical British diet; wheat and other cereal grains; milk and dairy products, including eggs; sugar; coffee and tea; chocolate; citrus, and alcohol. Two facts about these particular foods stand out.

One is that because their regular consumption is customary in Britain, they are surrounded by a dense and complex thicket of supporting social institutions and artefacts. Let us just consider the landscape of the typical British breakfast table. There is a coffee-pot or teapot in a hand-knit cosy, a stainless-steel toast-rack, egg-cups and special egg-spoons, a sugar bowl, a jam-pot or a crock of fancy marmalade, coffee or tea cups nesting in their saucers, cereal bowls, a milk jug, perhaps a cream pitcher. All these specialized, ritual objects testify to the traditional importance of the respective foods in the British way of life. In the kitchen area, we find an old-fashioned juice squeezer, – a relic of bygone days, now replaced by the nifty electric juicer, which also doubles as a coffee grinder, an electric percolator, an electric kettle, an egg-rack, a breadbox. Outside the door, there is a special bottle rack with a counter to let the milkman know how many pints are required — Britain is one of the few countries in the world where milkmen still do their daily rounds — and down the road we find the dairy, a bakery, the coffee shop, which also does a line in imported teas, and, of course, the omnipresent pub. And somewhere in outer space there lurk the marketing boards and product information bureaux. In view of the many interests vested in creating and maintaining this state of affairs, it would not be surprising to encounter widespread resistance to the idea that the traditional English breakfast, dear to the hearts of hoteliers, food and household gear manufacturers and sellers, is a feast of food allergens.

In addition to the many supporting social customs and their respective allergen-preparation-and-ingestion devices, the foods in the group of most commonly mentioned troublemakers also share the fact of being the most intensively and repetitively advertised. Since people eat these things every day, there is a huge market for them and hence considerable profits to be made by creating brand loyalties or, in the case of the product marketing boards, by encouraging increasing consumption. Thus magazine advertisements, posters on hoardings and on the sides of buses, bus shelters, and tube platforms, media commercials, coupons printed in the press or pushed through the letterbox, slogans, jingles, skits, competitions, items in packages and numerous other ploys all conspire to induce the public to consume more and more of their allergens. They are reminded to start their day with well-known brands of wheat cereal and instant coffee, to 'go to work on an egg', to 'drinka pinta milka day', and not to 'cheat on the cheese'. Self-indulgence in leering chocolate eclairs or mounded cream cakes is proclaimed as 'naughty but nice'. A child with butter melting in his mouth and a tender maiden tied to the railroad tracks who is saved from the jaws of fate by a gallant cup of tea prompt others to choose as they have been choosing for many years, while real oranges and lemons, gleaming from the passing buses, vie with their synthetic counterparts to provide the public with its daily Vitamin C. The advertisers draw on the teachings of motivational research[5] and sales figures show that the consuming public learn their lessons.

Both the social institutions surrounding the consumption of the leading food allergens and the massive support it receives from advertising promote a climate of opinion and practice which not only helps to create sufferers from food allergy, but also makes it difficult for people whose constitutional allergic tendency has succumbed to the onslaught of repetitive exposure to live normally in society once their allergy has come to light. As we shall see in subsequent chapters, the person who is allergic to common foods is multiply handicapped socially, more so than a person would be who was allergic only to uncommon foods. The cultural tradition of dietary staples means that they are extraordinarily hard to avoid unless one prepares and provides all one's own food from basic ingredients. In public eating places — restaurants, cafés, canteens, hospitals, airlines, buffet cars — and on social eating occasions, the vast majority of foods that are available are likely to contain at least one major food allergen. In addition to the restricted choice resulting from the omnipresence of the same few staples, the person allergic to common foods is also likely to encounter disbelief and resistance to the idea that his allergens can make him sick: 'No one is allergic to bread/milk/orange squash/tea/sugar, etc' he may be told. By contrast, if the allergen were an uncommon, unfamiliar food, such as kohlrabi, persimmons, or kumquats, people would probably not be surprised to hear that they were allergenic. Xenophobia manifests itself in many ways. Moreover, it is inconvenient for others, especially institutions, to be faced with the task of catering for someone with common food allergies. In some exceptionally rigid circumstances, exceptions may not be permitted and the unfortunate person who cannot eat what is served will be expected to go without. Blaming the victim also takes many forms.

The consequences to the sufferer of the coalition of powerful forces and vested interest at so many different levels can be very grave; the rest of this book deals with these consequences. In the next chapter we shall consider the symptoms which the survey respondents reported as a consequence of exposure to their allergens and in the following one the effects which their condition has upon their everyday lives.

4.

Symptoms

In this chapter we will consider the reactions that survey respondents reported experiencing when exposed to their allergens. Many of the symptoms that were mentioned are not the stuff of which orthodox allergy textbook lists of symptoms are made. In particular, as we shall see, a large proportion of the reactions described by members of the survey sample represented effects on the central nervous system, psychological functioning, and behaviour. Of all the findings about food allergy and chemical hypersensitivity, none is perhaps more contentious and controversial than the fact that the brain, mind, emotions and behaviour can be adversely affected by allergens.

Why there should be such enormous and widespread resistance to this idea is difficult to imagine. The resistance seems to represent an excellent example of a curious mental mechanism which I shall call the *kreplach phenomenon*. The name derives from an old joke about a little boy who had a phobia of kreplach, a Jewish dish consisting of a savoury paste filling in a kind of pasta shell, a bit like a ravioli. Whenever this boy encountered kreplach, he would let out a shriek and run from the room. One day his grandmother decided to try to eliminate his irrational fear of this perfectly harmless food. So she invited him into the kitchen to watch how it was made. he sat quietly as she demonstrated how she made the filling and mixed the dough for the pasta. He looked on with interest as she rolled out the dough and cut it into little sqares. He watched intently as she placed a bit of the filling in the centre of a square. He didn't bat an eyelid as she took the square that was to be the top and attached it to the first corner. He observed keenly as she attached the second corner. 'I see, Grandma,' he said as she attached the third corner. Then she attached the fourth corner, completing the piece. At this point the lad fled from the kitchen, screaming, 'Oi, kreplach!'

The emotional reaction of many who profess to be sceptical of the idea that particular substances can cause people to have mental symptoms is very similar to that of the little boy in the joke. The sceptics will assent to all the prior assumptions necessary to an acceptance of the proposition. They will cheerfully agree, for example, that of course drugs can affect the central nervous system, that drugs are chemicals, that individuals can have idiosyncratic adverse reactions to them or can develop side effects or toxicity at lower dose levels than it takes most people to do so, that foods consist of, contain, and are metabolized to other, chemicals, that the chemicals in foods affect many bodily tissues, that allergy is a tissue reaction, that the cerebral cortex is a tissue, that like other tissues the brain can react to external trauma — such as a blow to the head — by swelling and derangement or loss of function, that all the other tissues of the body are also known to react to the internal assault of allergens, and so on. But when a clinical ecologist puts all these prior assumptions together to form the concept of cerebral allergy, the sceptics holler, 'Oi, kreplach!' and flee, ostrich-like, back to the safety of their familiar prejudices, from where they ignore the well-designed, double-blind placebo controlled studies of the effects on the central nervous system (CNS) of food allergens and food metabolites that continue to appear in the literature.[1] People have known for centuries that foods can affect mental functioning, so the sceptics' reservations seem extremely retrograde, and their obstructiveness helps only to ensure that many people are deprived of the considerable benefits to be gained from treatment based on the rediscovery of this old truth.

Bearing these considerations in mind, let us examine the respondents' reports about the reactions provoked by their allergens.

Numbers of Types of Symptom

Like allergens, symptoms were analysed in the first instance according to categories. Women showed a much larger range of symptoms (1–28) than men (1–17) and also reported a higher average number of symptom types: 8.26 (S.D. 5.28) as against 5.95 (S.D. 3.67) for men.

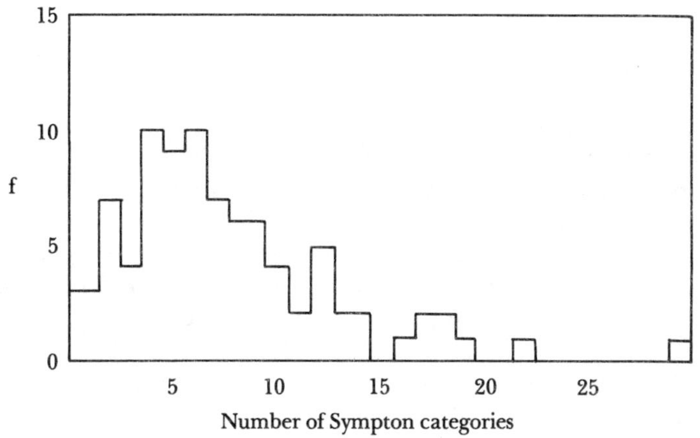

Figure 2.

A frequency histogram was plotted for the number of symptom categories reported per respondent. This graph is shown in Figure 2. As with the allergens, the distribution of symptoms shows an essentially trimodal pattern. The first group contains fourteen individuals with between one and three types of symptom, the second sixty three people with between four and fourteen types, and a third group contains eight with between sixteen and twenty eight types of symptom. In terms of the range of symptomatology, the three groups could be regarded as mildly, moderately, and severely affected by their allergic condition. In a later chapter we will consider the relation of these categories to the social limitations arising from the condition. Here we may look at some typical examples of the sorts of sufferers in each of the three categories.

Two Mildly Affected People

Charles M, a middle-aged physician, is allergic to mushrooms, which make his fingers and toes itch; thereafter the skin flakes and peels. Tomatoes produce itching and swelling of his hands, hives behind the ears, and ringing in the ears. He suspects fruit seeds of causing similar reactions to tomatoes.

Sylvia H, a trainee clinical psychologist in her early twenties, reports that chocolate and peanuts bring her out in spots, give her a headache, and a feeling of heat. Cigarette smoke also gives her a headache and coffee produces a racing heart. Bran and fibre also irritate her colon.

Two Moderately Affected People

Ted J, a twenty four year-old student, finds that fresh (but not canned) peaches give him watery eyes, a runny nose and an itchy mouth, which feels mildly inflamed. Some types of apple, consumed raw, produce itching and mouth inflammation. Traffic fumes give him a headache. He has a history of mild hay fever and up till the age of thirteen suffered from asthma. Cat fur, if inhaled, makes him wheezy even today and he cannot sleep in a room where a cat has been recently.

Roberta N, a secretary in her mid-thirties, develops an itchy rash on her face and neck after eating mushrooms. Tinned foods give her an upset stomach, headache and diarrhoea. Whisky and lager can make her irritable and aggressive. When tested for tea and egg she developed a throbbing of the face. Exposure to phenol leaves her unable to concentrate. Car fumes and Xerox photocopies give her a pain the left side of her neck and make her sleepy and unable to concentrate. When taking a particular contraceptive pill, she would be ill for about two and a half weeks almost every month, with fevers, a blotchy face, aching muscles, especially in her face, neck, left arm and chest. Roberta also suspects lettuce of giving her diarrhoea and finds that cooked cheese makes her feel sick.

Two Severely Affected People

Brian F, in his mid-fifties, holds a highly qualified professional post in local government in a city in the North of England. He is allergic to yeast and a wide variety of foods: corn, wheat, oats, rice, cane, runner bean, soya, potato, brassicas, carrot, onion, beet sugar, honey, peach, orange, grape, banana, apple, milk and egg-white. The only foods so far identified that he does not react to are pork, beef, lamb, chicken, pea, tomato and egg-yolk. His reactions to his allergens include one or more of the following symptoms: drowsiness, mental sluggishness, loss of memory, difficulty in expressing himself, depression, irritability, overreaction to events, physical weakness – particularly in the legs, a thick head, eyes out of focus, impaired hearing, catarrh, face sores, oedema, loss or gain of weight up to 5 lb (2.25 kg) in twelve hours, pulse varying from 38–76 beats per minute, pain in chest and elbows, itching of hips, forearms and anus, bowel distension, diarrhoea, gas and fluid from the bowel, sweating, feeling unnaturally cold, and prolonged sleep.

Andrea A, a middle-aged wife and mother, is allergic to wheat, corn, rye, oats, barley and rice, coffee and tea, alcohol, phenol and diesel fumes. After riding in a minibus, she was quite ill for several weeks, with a stomach ache, exhaustion, disorientation and slight depression. Her reactions to cereals take the form of a gradual build-up. For about five to ten days she has frequency of micturition, tension, irritability, swellings of hands, stomach and eyelids. Her eyes become very dry and the skin on the lids underneath becomes red and sore. Her insides feel all toxic. Her tongue is thickly coated and she starts to sweat heavily. She experiences palpitations, chronic fatigue, disorientation, confusion and a feeling of heaviness on her chest almost as though she were starting a chesty cold. Then any time from the fifth day onwards, depending on how concentrated the dose was, Andrea develops an acute depression that nothing will lift until the food is out of her system. She also has aches and pains all over her body and the constipation that normally troubles her becomes much worse.

The Symptoms Themselves
The frequencies with which the various types of symptoms were mentioned are shown in Table 11. It is clear from the table that symptoms commonly associated with allergy come at the top of the list and that symptoms which most people would probably not ordinarily associate with allergic reactions come towards the bottom. Thus the findings have a certain overall plausibility: they are about what might be expected.

Less immediately obvious is the high proportion of symptoms affecting the central nervous system (CNS), psychological functioning and behaviour. If all these symptoms are added together, the total comes to 40.09 per cent of all symptoms reported. The percentages of CNS, psychological and behavioural symptoms are marginally higher for men (42.02

Table 11: Frequency with which types of symptoms were reported
by survey respondents

Frequency	Symptom type
47	Migraine and headache
45	Respiratory
44	Abdominal
41	Skin lesions
31	Energy loss
30	Oedema and bloating
29	Bowel
27	Mental dullness and confusion
25	Skin sensations
24	Nausea and vomiting
23	Cardiovascular depression
22	Aggression and irritability
	Eyes
21	Vasomotor
20	Malaise
19	Joints and muscles
18	Clouded consciousness
12	Anxiety
11	Hyperactivity
10	Genitourinary
9	Tension
8	Hypersomnia
7	Speech and reading difficulties
	Weepiness
	Social withdrawal
	Ears and hearing
5	Menstrual difficulties
	Insomnia
	Weakness
4	Prostration
	Addictive behaviour
	Foul taste in mouth
	Psychotic symptoms
	Depersonalization–derealization
3	Mood swings
	Neuralgia
2	Bruising
	Nightmares
	Extreme hunger and thirst
	Chinese Restaurant Syndrome
	Shock

Table 11: continued

Frequency	Symptom type
1	Enuresis
	Obsessions
	Obesity
	'Hysterics'
	Photophobia
	Broken nails
	Arthritic nodules
	Travel sickness
	Nasal polyps
	Phobia
	Swollen glands
	Behaviour problems

per cent) than for women (39.66 per cent). The findings of such a high proportion of 'mental' symptoms is definitely not what most orthodox allergy textbooks would lead us to expect. However, in addition to the physically-oriented allergy literature, which emphasizes respiratory difficulties such as asthma, bronchitis and hay fever, skin complaints such as eczema and dermatitis and abdominal problems such as diarrhoea, abdominal pain, and the like, there is also a fairly extensive minor literature on allergy of the nervous system,[2] in the light of which these findings would not be in the least surprising. What *is* surprising, on the other hand, is that allergy is so little appreciated, either by the general public or by mental-health professionals, including medically-qualified psychiatrists who, whatever their ultimate orientation, have studied organic psychiatry in some depth as part of their medical training. The failure to recognize allergy as a potential factor in the causation of mental disorder probably arises from the fact that it is not included as a topic in standard works on the subject, such as Lishman's otherwise very comprehensive textbook.[3]

This lack of recognition accorded to the possible role of food intolerance in the genesis of some people's mental distress and disorder has a number of unfortunate consequences. One is that sufferers from unrecognized food-induced psychopathology are treated as if they were suffering from so-called functional disorders and continue to be exposed to the sources of their difficulties as they are treated with drugs which, if they work at all, do so merely by suppressing the symptoms. A more sinister consequence awaits those who are aware of the role which foods play in their mental state. It is entirely possible that the sufferer's view that this, that or the other common food is contributing to his or her illness may be dismissed out of hand as a hypochondriacal or paranoid fantasy instead of being taken seriously. If such people were to be hospitalized for treatment, they would probably find it extraordinarily difficult to escape contact with the most likely causes of their trouble, as we will see in the following section.

Table 12: Dietary substances associated with depression in twenty-three respondents

Frequency	%	Substance	Frequency	%	Substance
12	52.17	Wheat	2	8.70	Cream
8	34.78	Cheese			Butter
7	30.43	Coffee			Lamb
		Milk			Beef
		Egg			Pork
6	26.09	Chocolate/			Chicken
		cocoa			Peanuts
		Alcohol			Turkey
5	21.74	Tea	1	4.35	Runner bean
		Cane Sugar			Beet sugar
4	17.39	Citrus			Peach
		Corn			Trifle
		Carrot			Pork sausage
		Grape			Gluten-free
		Banana			flour
		Oats			Margerine
		Rye			Marmite
3	13.04	Rice			Apple-juice
		Soya			concentrate
		Potato			Soft drinks
		Onion family			Coconut
		Yeast			Smoked foods
		Barley			Butter beans
		Tinned foods			Tomato
2	8.70	Brassicas			Parnsip
		Honey			Lettuce
		Apple			Blackcurrant
		Instant/			Shellfish
		packet foods			Tap water
		Ice-cream			Bacon

Environmental Precipitants of Depression

The dietary substances that the twenty three respondents who reported depression as a symptom of their allergic reactions named as precipitants of their depressive states were analysed and frequency counts obtained. These findings appear in Table 12.

We can readily see from the table that many respondents appear to experience similar effects from similar causes. Over half the group reported depressive effects from wheat, over thirty per cent from cheese, coffee, milk and egg, and over twenty per cent from tea, alcohol, chocolate or cocoa, and cane sugar. The remaining common grains – corns, oats, rye, rice and barley — and common foods such as citrus, carrot, grape and banana, were also mentioned by a substantial percentage of the depressed subsample. While the numbers are too small to be more than suggestive, the findings do indicate that people's experiences in this department are not merely idiosyncratic and deserve further investigation in a larger sample.[4] Meanwhile, it seems evident that the typical high-cereal, milk, and egg-based hospital diet, with only coffee, tea and orange juice or squash provided as beverages on the menu is likely to be disastrous for a considerable proportion of sufferers from food-induced depression.

One question which may be raised in considering these findings is: how severe are the depressive states induced by foods? Although it was not possible to tell in all cases whether a clinical depressive illness or a more 'normal' depressed mood state was meant, it was clear that many respondents had been treated for clinical depressions. Some had been hospitalized, whilst others attended as out-patients. But our data are not sufficient to establish anything further than that some people appear to suffer from clinical depressive illnesses that are apparently precipitated by foods and that the problem urgently requires further study.

These findings are less revolutionary than they might at first appear to some who are only acquainted with recent theories of the aetiology of depression. They gain a certain perspective in the light of medical history. In neo-classical medicine, as transmitted to the English-speaking world in Burton's *Anatomy of Melancholy*, which appeared in 1621,[5] certain foods were regarded as bad for people possessed of a melancholic tendency. These included a number which appear on the list of foods indicated by the survey respondents in the years 1979-80: milk and milk products, alcohol, sugar (which in the seventeenth century was a spice rather than a staple food), carrot, oats, beans, onion, rye, honey, apple, beef, pork and parsnip; and also 'an infinite number of compound, artificial, made dishes, of which our cooks afford us a great variety, as tailors do fashions in apparel'. Of course, the basis for excluding foods was the ancient theory of humoral pathology and conventional notions about the propensity of various foods to engender melancholy humours in the body. Foods which were thought to be inclined to leave residues, or 'dregs', from which black bile was made, were proscribed. Although the theory is now discredited, and although on some points the ancients gave advice which would be viewed askance today – for example, Burton cites authorities who recommend white wheaten bread, with all the impurities removed – the overlap between the present-day empirical reports of sufferers and the ancient recommendations is probably less than entirely coincidental. The ancients were in just as good a position as the moderns to observe the effects of particular foods on their well-being and their observations probably provided the basis for the theory, which was then elaborated.

Where the moderns differ is in possessing techniques for the elucidation of mechanisms by which observable correlations between foods and mental states could be brought about. In February 1979, there appeared in the *Lancet* an editorial on food allergy[6] which workers in the field, battling against entrenched institutional resistance to ecological ideas, regard with some gratitude as one of the first official acknowledgements by the conservative British medical establishment that food allergy exists and is worthy of the attention of clinical and research workers in many branches of medicine. The editorial refers to three contemporary sources of the idea that certain foods may induce mental disorder (Mackarness; Dohan; Kety[7]), alludes to Burton, and notes that the idea now receives some support from the work of Hemmings,[8] who has shown that in the rat, whose metabolism is not dissimilar from that of humans, up to half of the intake of milk and wheat protein is not broken down into amino acids and small peptide molecules in the gut, but is absorbed in the form of large molecules and can be traced directly to the brain. These large breakdown products can retain the antigenic properties of the parent substances from which they are formed.

But even if an individual is not allergic to milk and wheat, these foods may exert psychonoxious effects by other means. Independent research by Zioudrou and her co-workers[9] has shown that certain proteins in milk and wheat are broken down in the course of digestion to substances which behave like naturally-occurring opiate molecules called endorphins and can attach to the appropriate receptors in the brain, where they can affect mental functioning. These food-derived molecules have been named exorphins. Their possible role in normal and abnormal mental functioning is currently being debated.

Although these findings have been put forward in the context of providing an explanation for the observations on the role of milk and wheat in schizophrenia, there seems to be no good reason why these or similar mechanisms should not be involved in the genesis of at least some people's depressions. In any event, it now seems to have been established beyond any reasonable doubt that residues of certain foodstuffs can enter the brain in antigenically recognizable form and that breakdown products of these same foods are capable of chemical activity within the central nervous system. The pathophysiological differences between the major forms of so-called 'functional' mental disorder may turn out to be due to corresponding differences in the affected individual's genetically-determined propensity to derangement of particular neurotransmitter systems. The findings that antidepressant drugs can block brain histamine receptors,[10] whereas antipsychotic drugs — and high-dose Vitamin C, which has been found to have a similar action[11] — block dopamine receptors is consistent with this notion. In addition, differences in the availability of hormone-like substances called prostaglandins[12] are also likely to be involved.

Although the final answer has not yet been worked out in detail, it is fairly clear, even in the present imperfect state of knowledge, that the neurochemistry and physiology of the major mental disorders are too complex to be reduced to a simple matter of food A causing pathology B, with nothing else happening in between. Account must also be taken of the genetically determined individual differences that predispose to particular sorts of biochemical disturbance[13] and other trigger factors that determine why eating the food at one point in time precipitates problems that have probably not appeared on every single occasion that the food has been consumed.

Immunological as well as biochemical individuality must play a role.[14] But it now appears virtually certain that intolerance of particular foods does contribute in important ways to some people's mental disturbances. This possibility is not yet taken sufficiently seriously by the majority of British health workers, including those who plan hospital menus.

Table 13: Non-dietary substances associated with depression in four respondents

Frequency	Substance
2	Phenol
	Diesel fumes
1	Ethanol
	Paint
	Stain
	Tar
	Glycerine
	Dry cleaning fluid
	Gas
	Petrol
	Nylon
	Plastic
	Detergent
	Antiseptic
	Candles
	Shampoo
	Chlorine
	Perfume
	New suede
	Hay

In addition to foods, respondents also reported non-dietary environmental precipitants of depression. These substances are shown in Table 13. In all, four respondents reported inhalants, so the totals are lower than in the previous table. The numbers are too small to be more than indicative, but it does appear from the table that a wide range of individual substances is involved, chemicals and natural substances alike, and that chemicals comprise the larger category. It may be that there is no traditional lore about the effects of inhalants in depression because in the distant past when traditions were formed, the environment was not ubiquitously contaminated with chemical residues as it is now. In any case, the possibility that inhalant sensitivity can make people feel depressed is one which certainly requires further study in a larger sample.

The importance of environmental precipitants of CNS disorders will become more apparent in the next section, which deals with disorders that are even more prevalent than depression.

Environmental Precipitants of Headache and Migraine
Since migraine and headache were the most frequently reported symptoms, it is worth while examining the foods and other substances which respondents mentioned as precipitants. These findings are shown in Table 14. Many of the same foods appear at the top of this list as we saw at the top of the list of foods associated with depression, but they are in a somewhat different order. This finding suggests that the main dietary staples are the foods most likely to precipitate common mental symptoms but that the particular form which the symptoms assume depends upon the biochemical and immunological individuality of the sufferer.

How reliable are these findings? Since it was impossible, under the conditions of the study, to ask respondents to fill in the questionnaire twice, we may perhaps best answer this question by comparing the present results with others previously reported in the literature. At the time the data-collection phase of our study was nearing completion, Hanington[15] published her findings about the relative frequencies of dietary precipitants in a series of 500 migraine sufferers seen in her practice. Because her categories are somewhat different from the ones used in the present study, our data have been regrouped in order to make them more comparable with hers. These comparative figures are shown in Table 15.

Several facts emerge from the table. First, Hanington's patients do not appear to have mentioned wheat and wheat products, whereas over twenty five per cent of the present group identified it as a precipitant of their headaches and migraines. The difference may result from the fact that in the present study migrainous and non-migrainous headaches were grouped together in the same symptom category. Another difference is that more of Hanington's respondents reported chocolate, cheese and dairy foods, fatty and fried foods and meat as

Table 14: Dietary substances associated with migraine and headache in forty seven respondents

Frequency	Substance	Frequency	Substance
16	Chocolate	1	Millet
15	Alcohol		Buckwheat
13	Coffee		Yeast
12	Wheat and wheat		Shellfish
	products		Celery
11	Cheese		Parnsip
10	Cows' milk		Confectionery
8	Tea		Courgettes
7	Citrus, esp. oranges		Melon
6	Corn		Cucumber
	Peanut		Margerine
5	Eggs		Marmite
	Rice		Apple-juice
4	Barley		concentrate
	Oats		Camp coffee
	Onion family		Preservatives
	Ice-cream		Lucozade
	Cream		Smoked foods
	Butter		Mushrooms
	Banana		Beef
	Cane sugar		Beans
3	Brassicas		Perrier water
	Pork		Fatty foods
	Chicken		Coconut
	Nuts		Baked beans
	Rye		Foods containing
	Packet foods		large amounts of
2	Animal fats		calcium
	Lettuce		Butter beans
	Processed meats		Lentils
	Tomatoes		Watercress
	Fish		Cherry
	Peas		Peach
	Carrot		Apricot
	Grape		Pineapple
	Raisin		Currant
	Glucose		Gooseberry
	Sweet biscuits		Peppercorn
	Shortbread		Chicory
	Apples		Coriander
	Fried fish		Lactose

Table 14: continued

Frequency Substance	Frequency Substance
Plums	Mutton
Tinned foods	MSG
Squash and soft	
drinks	
Broad beans	
Soya	

precipitants, whereas more of the present group reported alcohol, vegetables, tea and coffee. Seafood was reported about equally often in both groups. Third, although the percentages differ, the rank order of the dietary precipitants identified by both groups is highly similar. The Spearman rank order correlation coefficient, a measure of the degree to which observations occur in the same order in different groups, was + 0.671, which is high, positive, and significant at the five per cent level. Considering the widely differing circumstances under which the two studies were conducted, the high degree of similarity between the results should give us some confidence in the present findings. In this context, it is also encouraging that in her studies of sixty migraine patients attending a hospital clinic, the most common foods implicated were all mentioned by our own respondents. Grant's figures for her series were:

wheat (78 per cent)	tea and coffee (40 per cent each)
orange (65 per cent)	chocolate and milk (37 per cent each)
eggs (45 per cent)	corn, cane sugar, yeast (33 per cent each).[16]

Grant's finding that wheat was a common source of difficulty in migraine sufferers is, like our own result, discrepant with Hanington's results. It seems likely that the discrepancy may arise not only through the differences between the samples mentioned earlier but also through differences in methods of allergen detection. Hanington does not specify how her respondents arrived at their knowledge of which foods affected them adversely, but it seems unlikely that it was by means of the application of ecological methods. With the exception of coffee

Table 15: Comparative frequency of foods associated with migraine
in two studies

	Hanington 1980	Present study (1979–80)
	n = 500	n = 47
Food	%	%
Chocolate	75	34
Cheese and dairy*	48	34
Citrus	30	17
Alcohol	25	32
Fatty fried foods	18	6
Vegetables, esp. onions	18	21
Tea and coffee	14	32
Meat esp. pork	14	11
Seafood	10	11

*including eggs

and tea, the foods her respondents mentioned tend not to be
consumed regularly at every meal and so might be likely to
cause difficulties after acute exposure — such foods are more
readily detectable than masked allergens. But wheat, by
contrast, would tend to cause its noxious effects in migraine
sufferers by means of masking and would thus require
ecological methods for its detection. As we will see in the
chapters on help seeking and self-help, these are precisely the
methods most commonly adopted by members of the present
sample for the detection of their culprits, and they are also the
methods employed by Grant with her patients. The similarity of
methods is probably the main reason for the incrimination of
foods such as cereal grains, yeast and sugar by the two groups of
sufferers.

In addition to dietary precipitants, a number of survey
respondents also identified chemicals and other inhalants as
causes of their headaches. The chemically-sensitive were a
minority: thirty respondents named only foods as precipitants,
five both foods and inhalants, four inhalants only, and eight did
not specify the cause of their migraines and headaches. Thus of
those who specified, about a quarter were troubled by
inhalants. Although these people are a minority, they are an
important one, because hypersensitivity to inhalants is not
widely regarded as a common cause of headaches, possibly
because the traditional views of migraine and headaches were
formed at a time when the environment was not polluted by the

Table 16: Non-dietary precipitants of migraine and headache
reported by survey respondents

Frequency	Precipitant
3	Paraffin heaters
	Paint fumes
	Petrol fumes
2	North Sea gas
	Perfumes
	Diesel fumes
	Tobacco fumes
1	Air freshener
	White spirit
	Phenol
	Ethanol
	Stain
	Tar
	Glycerine
	Dry-cleaning fluid
	Shampoo
	Chlorine detergents
	Antiseptics
	Butane
	Hay

inhalants that contemporary respondents indict. These
inhalants are listed in Table 16.

Of all the inhalants mentioned, only one (hay) is not a
chemical. Hydrocarbon fumes were by far the most common
type of substance causing difficulty. The ubiquitousness of the
most common fumes in ordinary urban environments, both
indoor and outdoor, and their variety, suggest that people who
are hypersensitive to them will probably encounter a host of
difficult problems in trying to avoid contact with them and that
these problems will differ in important ways from those
inherent in avoiding unsafe foods. We will return to this point
in the chapter on limitations arising from hypersensitivity.

Environmental Precipitants of Psychotic Symptoms
Since only four respondents mentioned psychotic symptoms
such as delusions, ideas of reference, and chaotic or irrational
thoughts, the results of the following analysis are hardly more
than indicative. However, in view of the degree of agreement

Table 17: Environmental precipitant of psychotic symptoms
mentioned by four respondents

Frequency	Substance
4	Wheat
3	Carrot
	Chocolate/cocoa
2	Coffee
	Alcohol
	Banana
	Cheese
	Ice-cream
	Corn
	Egg
	Yeast
	Confectionery/sugar
1	Citrus
	Pork sausage
	Packet/instant foods
	Bacon
	Rye
	Barley
	Peanut
	Oats
	Rice
	Chicken
	Shellfish
	Pea
	Tomato
	Celery
	Parsnip
	Grape
	Lettuce
	Onion
	Tinned foods
	Smoked foods
	Honey
	Butter beans
	House dust

between four completely independent respondents, the findings, skeletal as they are, nonetheless seemed worth reporting. They are shown in Table 17. The most striking finding is that 100 per cent of respondents named wheat as a source of trouble, and that fifty per cent named cheese and ice-cream – both milk products – and coffee. These findings are consistent with the studies of the metabolism of proteins in wheat and milk that were mentioned earlier and also with other research on the psychonoxious effects of coffee.[17] The high proportion of people mentioning chocolate and sugar is consistent with findings about anomalies of carbohydrate metabolism in various forms of mental illness, including schizophrenia.[18] Why carrot should be mentioned so frequently is not clear, but it certainly suggests that further study of dietary factors in major mental disorders might uncover some important and unsuspected hazards in common foods.

Table 18: Environmental precipitants of hyperactivity in eleven respondents

Frequency	Substance
10	Artificial flavours
9	Artificial colours
8	Preservatives
7	Cows' milk
5	Wheat and wheat products
4	Sugar
	Jam and confectionery
3	Grape/raisin
	Rice
	Rye
	Barley
	Oats
	Millet
2	Cheese
	Butter
	Chocolate
	Fruit drinks
	Banana
	Hair-spray
1	Red wine
	Egg
	Dried beans
	Peas
	Runner beans
	Citrus
	Yeast
	Gluten
	Onion

Chemical inhalants were not implicated by these four respondents as causing psychotic symptoms, but house dust was. In any event, it is clear that people with food-related psychotic symptoms would be at a serious disadvantage if exposed to hospital catering.

Environmental Precipitants of Hyperactivity
The dietary and other precipitants that respondents mentioned in connection with hyperactive behaviour problems are shown in Table 18.

Three features of the findings require commentary. First, the fact that artificial food additives head the list is consistent with Feingold's hypothesis[19] that these substances play an important role in many cases of hyperactivity. However, it is also clear from the differences in numbers of mothers reporting problems with these substances in their offspring — and, in some cases, themselves — that all affected individuals are not affected in a uniform manner. Second, the fact that many foods are also mentioned, in particular cow's milk, wheat and foods containing large amounts of sugar, suggest that for many affected children food allergy or intolerance also plays a part. A number of investigators have provided evidence that bears out this point.[20] Third, the fact that two individuals reported an exacerbation upon exposure to hair-spray indicates chemical hypersensitivity as a factor in some hyperactive individuals.

Multiple sensitivities such as these have previously been reported to cause childhood activity associated with many somatic symptoms. Mandell[21] reported the case of Laura Belanger, a bright young schoolgirl with learning disabilities who was found upon sublingual testing to react to a variety of foods, food additives and contaminants, and inhalants, both synthetic and natural. His report includes samples of the girl's handwriting both under normal conditions and after acute exposure to her environmental precipitants. After exposure, letter reversals were observed and she even misspelled her own name. After a massive housecleaning campaign and the institution of appropriate dietary measures, Laura was reported to have settled at school.

It is clear both from the present findings and from cases such as Laura's that food additives are not the only environmental precipitants in some, probably many, cases of hyperactivity. This point has implications both for the use of dietary treatment with hyperactive children and for research on the efficacy of such treatment. As Forman has noted in his discussion of Mandell's views on the Feingold diet,[22] there is the danger that if excluding additives alone doesn't work, the parents may conclude that environmental precipitants are not responsible for the child's behaviour disorder and abandon the search prematurely. Second, research on the problem, which has focused almost exclusively on trying to establish — or, it often seems, to disprove — the efficacy of the Feingold diet may fall into the same trap. Because research protocols normally specify that all subjects must receive uniform treatment, and because the treatment under investigation — the exclusion of certain classes of dietary additives — represents only a very limited approach to a problem which, as we have seen, can have a much wider network of environmental ramifications, the conclusions that can be drawn in many cases from the studies in existence are bound to be misleading. If, on the other hand, researchers were prepared to investigate the effects of elimination regimens worked out by a clinical ecologist for each individual child, a very different picture of the role of environmental factors in the genesis of hyperactivity might in due course grace the walls of the establishment.

It is a dreadful pity that so much research effort and energy has been devoted by so many people all over the world to investigating one particular and incomplete approach to the baffling problem of hyperactivity and that so little has been expended upon this potentially more high-powered method of tackling the condition. It is also a great shame that a wider awareness of hypersensitivity to foods as a possible cause of behaviour disturbance has not coloured the research on additives to date. In the apparent absence of such awareness, investigators have committed a number of major methodological blunders, such as designing a 'control' diet which excludes a great number of common food allergens and using chocolate, a potent and common allergen, as a *placebo* in challenge studies.[23] Understandably, as a result, the studies have failed to yield clear-cut findings and it is to be feared that the Establishment may lose interest and shelve the topic before dietary and other nutritional methods, such as the use of essential fatty acids and vitamin and mineral supplements,[24] have been given a fair chance to show what they can do.

The sorry outcome of such a state of affairs will be that

potentially noxious additives remain firmly entrenched in the food supply and those who wish to avoid them will be hampered by the fact that information about their particular identity will continue to be withheld from the label — with full Government assent. In a recent report in the *Sunday Times*, the company secretary of Schweppes, which had decided not to inform the public which of its soft-drink products contain the much-investigated dye, tartrazine, was quoted as saying, 'We are not so arrogant as to think that we can make these health assessments ourselves. We rely on the advice of government committees.'[25] In the same article, a spokesman for the Food and Drink Industries Council was quoted as saying that, 'In France, where they have more detailed labelling, scare stories have stopped people from buying food which contains additives. We don't want that to happen here.' Of course they don't! We have here further evidence of the concert of powerful vested interests that conspire not only to contribute to the creation of environmental casualties but also, having created them, to make it difficult for them to avoid further damage.

Meanwhile, if dietary approaches are not considered seriously and knowledgeably and as a result are dismissed prematurely, another outcome will be that many children will end up having their hyperactive behaviour 'managed' by centrally-acting stimulant drugs (which may themselves contain artificial colours and sugar coatings, not to mention other possible allergens as fillers). Others will be given neuroleptic drugs. And a proportion of these children, whose central nervous systems are still developing, will develop side-effects. The list of unwanted complications which these drugs — principally methylphenidate, dextroamphetamine sulphate, and chlorpromazine — have been reported to have produced in young children does not make pleasant reading. They include depression of growth; hallucinosis; excitement followed by catatonic withdrawal; tics; dyskinesias (abnormal grimacing, lip-smacking movements, twisting of head and limbs, and the like); decreased appetite; stomach-aches; regressive, dependent behaviour; and overt psychosis.[26] While these reactions appear to be uncommon, the fact that they occur at all is a matter of concern. By contrast, no harm has ever been reported in the medical literature to have befallen children as a consequence of *not* consuming tartrazine, erythrosine, BHA (butylated hydroyanisole), BHT (butylated hydroxytoluene) and other additives.

Whichever way we look at it, someone stands to make a profit from the widespread failure to consider the role of environmental precipitants in the aetiology of hyperactive behaviour in children. In the next chapter we shall consider, among other things, the experiences of parents of such children when seeking medical help with the problem.

5.

Help-Seeking

The survey questionnaire included two questions about people's efforts to find outside help for their condition. These were:

1   Have you sought medical attention for these problems? If so, what was done about them by way of investigation and treatment, and how effective was/is the treatment?
2   Have you sought help from people other than doctors? If so, who, and with what outcome?

In this chapter we will examine respondents' replies to these questions. Let us consider medical help-seeking first.

Medical Help-seeking
The majority of respondents reported having sought medical attention for their condition. Only eight, or 9.41 per cent of the sample, reported not having seen a doctor. Three of these were themselves professionally qualified – one a doctor, one a nurse and one a psychologist. However, the doctor, Mike P, whom we met in Chapter 2, reported that he had several times been hospitalized with severe allergic reactions, so that although he did not need to seek medical assistance in obtaining a diagnosis, he has needed emergency medical aid. One of the other respondents who said he had not sought help was a coeliac, who presumably had contact with doctors at some stage of his life in

order to get his diagnosis. He gave as his reason for not seeking help that 'nothing can be done'. Thus whether or not they had actually consulted a doctor with a view to obtaining relief, very few respondents got by without some form of medical attention for their condition at some stage of their lives.

Table 19: Sources of medical attention mentioned by survey respondents

Source	f	%
GP	74	87.06
Hospital investigations	22	25.88
Clinical ecologist	21	24.71
Conventional allergy clinic	16	18.82
Physician-type unspecified	13	15.29
Psychiatrist	8	9.41
Other private doctor using some clinical ecology methods	6	7.06
Dermatologist	3	3.53
Surgeon	3	3.53
ENT specialist	2	2.35
Endocrinologist	2	2.35
Paediatrician	2	2.35
Neurologist	1	1.18
Gastroenterologist	1	1.18
Gynaecologist	1	1.18
Occupational health physician	1	1.18
No medical help sought	8	9.41

The range of doctors and medical departments mentioned was extensive. The findings are shown in Table 19, where it will be seen that the total adds up to considerably more than eighty five, because the majority who saw a doctor saw more than one. Several facts about the table are in need of comment. One is that the proportion of respondents who reported consulting a clinical ecologist is undoubtedly much higher than in the general population of allergic people. This atypical finding results immediately from the method of recruiting respondents: one group belonged to a self-help club organized for his former patients by a clinical ecologist and another group were members of the country's leading information service for sufferers, which, among other things, provides people with information about the availability of clinical ecology services. This incidental result is useful, since it will permit us to compare the outcome of clinical ecology treatment to that of conventional medicine and alternative medical treatments on the basis of a reasonable number of instances.

Second, although allergists represented the largest category of orthodox medical specialist that was named, the total number of respondents who were sent to practitioners in other specialities is more than twice as large. This finding suggests that the allergic nature of many people's problems may not be readily recognized at primary-care level, with consequent inefficiency in the deployment of scarce medical resources. Many respondents said that the hypothesis of allergy was suggested only after a large number of other possible causes had been excluded. Sometimes the process of exclusion required in-patient investigations lasting several weeks, at untold cost to the NHS and the taxpayer, and at the cost of much aggravation for the patient.

From respondents' accounts, it appeared, broadly, that GPs were more likely to recognize dermatological and acute respiratory difficulties such as asthma and hay fever as allergic than to appreciate the possibility of an environmental aetiology in central nervous system, rheumatological and multisymptomatic disorders. One exception was 'coffee nerves', which appeared to be readily recognizable and could be dealt with satisfactorily by appropriate advice at GP level.

Multiple specialist consultation seemed to be the rule amongst those who consulted specialists, a finding which again emphasizes the economic inefficiency of the situation. One woman with affected children, for example, wrote that she had taken them to ten different practitioners of the same speciality – all in vain. Others did not go into detail but declared that it would take many pages to chronicle their efforts to find relief. But some did recount their help-seeking histories in detail and it is instructive to consider a few of these.

Reg R

Reg R, a middle-aged specialist industrial worker, suffers from allergies to water, inhalants and numerous foods. The food allergies seem to affect his gut and nervous system; water irritates his skin, sometimes severely enough to cause muscle spasm and collapse, and the inhalants, whether organic, inorganic or synthetic, cause him respiratory problems. His job involves exposure to metal dusts and soap dust. After one particularly severe collapse, apparently precipitated by foods, he sought help from a private clinic, where homoeopathy, acupuncture, vitamin and dietary treatments were tried and blood tests revealed that he had a hypoglycaemic tendency. But he wasn't much better as a result. Thereafter, feeling he was getting nowhere, he tried to interest the occupational health doctors at his job in sorting out his occupational inhalant problems. Nothing came of his efforts. Then his GP referred him to a skin specialist locally, since he had by this time developed mild psoriasis. After numerous fruitless visits and treatments, ranging from iron tablets to aqueous cream to advice not to wash, he was referred on to a specialist skin hospital and was eventually admitted for a four-day in-patient stay. There Reg endured blood, stool and urine tests before seeing the consultant, who, hearing that Reg did not show visible wheals or skin reactions, told him there was nothing he could do. Reg left within the hour.

Thereafter, he developed persistent diarrhoea, a sore anus, and a generally rundown feeling. he was sent to see a surgeon, again with no outcome. Eventually, after he had seen a total of four specialists, his local skin consultant sent him to a clinical ecologist, who diagnosed his allergies to foods, coffee, tea, moulds and house dust and prescribed a regimen of vitamins and minerals that enabled him to return to a normal diet without diarrhoea. At the time of his report, the water allergy was still under investigation by the clinical ecologist.

Barbara G
Barbara G, a young language teacher, attached to her questionnaire a supplementary chart 24-in (610 mm) long describing a six-year history of problems, diagnoses, treatments, and her assessments of their effectiveness. There are fifteen problems recorded, most of them multiple. The first episode, of depersonalization and abdominal pain, was diagnosed by Barbara's GP as food poisoning and overwork. He prescribed her some medicine for the pain and a week's rest. The medicine helped, she said, but the week off didn't. The following month she appeared again, complaining of depersonalization, fear and irregular periods. This state was put down to her missing her routine after the week off, which coincided with the end of the academic year. She was assured that it would all settle when she returned to her course and

nothing was done about it. She continued to suffer. When the new term started and the depersonalization continued, Barbara was told she was sufferng from tension and anxiety and possible epilepsy (which in itself is enough to make many people tense and anxious) and was given Valium, which she found fairly effective. She was to return to the doctor to be sent for investigations for epilepsy if the problem didn't settle, but she was too frightened by the prospect to go back to see him. The following summer, she returned with a headache, fever and severe abdominal pain, which received a diagnosis of a virus and urinary tract infection. Nothing was done about the virus for the first few days, then paracetemol was prescribed, with no effect. Repeated testing of urine samples eventually led to the prescription of antibiotics, which eventually sorted out the urinary tract infection. The following summer, after moving house and starting a new job, Barbara again appeared with depersonalization, fear and lethargy. These were attributed to settling down and overwork. Again Valium was given with some benefit.

The next episode in Barbara's troubles involved difficulties with her ears and resulted in an ear operation, which left her feeling depersonalized, depressed, fearful and generally ill. She was sent to another specialist with a provisional diagnosis of migraine, treated with a tonic, a standard migraine remedy, and a month off work. These interventions were not very effective. The following year, she presented herself yet again — this time with lethargy, loss of appetite, weight gain, abdominal pain and feeling sick. Thyroid underfunctioning was suspected, but when blood tests proved negative Barbara's provisional diagnosis was changed to endogenous depression. Valium and antidepressants were prescribed; they worked for a few months.

When the drugs ceased to be effective after several months, Barbara reappeared in the surgery and was despatched to see a psychiatrist. He diagnosed anxiety and depersonalization, prescribed Valium, and sent Barbara for an EEG, which turned out to be inconclusive. The Valium had little effect, so two months later he added an antidepressant and Barbara improved. A further EEG, done at this time, was normal. Next Barbara was sent to a psychologist for relaxation training and behaviour therapy. Taken in conjunction with drugs, these interventions were helpful at first. Further behaviour therapy, however, failed to have much impact. Finally, another psychologist took over and Barbara's story took a major turn.

Though not a clinical ecologist (because the Society for Clinical Ecology restricts membership to those who are medically qualified), the psychologist used a range of ecological methods. Suspecting food allergy as the main cause of her troubles, he asked Barbara to keep records of her diet, mood, and levels of tension and energy. He arranged for a glucose tolerance test to be conducted and this revealed that Barbara was suffering from reactive hypoglycaemia. The psychologist advised her to adopt an antihypoglycaemia diet, helped her to identify her particular food allergens, encouraged her to read widely about her problem, and completely transformed her from a misunderstood misery to a 'different person'.

In both cases, a happy outcome only became possible when the allergic nature of the problem was recognized and clinical ecology methods were applied. This was true whether the clinician involved was actually a Clinical Ecologist or not; as long as the right questions were asked, the credentials of the person asking them was not a crucial factor. Indeed, as we shall see in a later chapter, many respondents were able to apply the concepts and techniques of clinical ecology by themselves, without benefit of firsthand contact with a relevant practitioner. The fact that many cases of allergy are amenable to self-diagnosis and self-treatment is one of the few saving graces of the condition and we shall look into people's self-help practices in the next chapter. But now we need to consider the care which respondents reported receiving from their medical advisors. In the discussion that follows, conventional medical measures will be distinguished from clinical ecology and alternative medicine measures in order to permit a broad comparison of their overall effectiveness, as judged by the recipients, to be made. Let us consider investigations first.

Investigations

Respondents mentioned a wide variety of investigations they had received from their GPs, consultants in various medical specialities, and other sources. Most who reported having any investigations said that they had had many, either for the same or for different sets of symptoms. Because patients are often not given full details about what assays are performed upon blood samples taken from them, they often reported their investigations in a generic way, e.g. 'blood tests', 'skin tests', and sometimes just plain 'investigations'. However, the data are sufficient to indicate trends in respondents' experiences.

In the analyses that follow, investigations and other treatments will be grouped under three broad headings: 'conventional', which refers to non-ecological approaches available within the NHS; 'clinical ecology', whether obtained under the NHS or privately; and 'alternative', which includes homoeopathy and other non-conventional approaches – all, with the exception of homoeopathy, unavailable under the NHS. The aim of this classification is to permit a broad comparison of the various sources of assistance available to members of the survey sample.

Table 20:   Investigations mentioned by survey respondents

Type of investigation	f
Conventional	
Allergy tests–unspecified	4
Skin tests (hospital)	11
Blood tests (hospital)	9
Other physical investigations	17
Clinical ecology	
Allergy tests unspecified	3
Skin tests	5
Pulse test	2
Provocative tests	3
Sublingual testing	2
Glucose tolerance test	1
Elimination diet (as investigative procedure)	8
Fast	1
Diet and symptom diary	5
Alternative medicine	
Glucose tolerance test	2
Other	
Blood tests–private laboratory	5

The frequency of the different sorts of investigations that were mentioned are shown in Table 20. The first thing that stands out is that relatively few respondents reported having been investigated for allergy. Only one of the blood tests reported was clearly recognizable as an immunological investigation ('it showed no antibody'). Second, it appears from respondents' reports that conventional allergy tests are more restricted in their range than clinical ecology investigations, which included elimination diets as a means of finding out about the effects of particular types of food as well as a method of avoiding symptoms from contact with identified precipitants. Although elimination diets are used as an investigation technique in some allergy clinics, no respondents reported having been given one at a conventional clinic. The skin tests reported under the heading of clinical ecology investigations were of two types: intradermal prick tests to identify allergens and skin titration tests to determine the level of dilution required for neutralization drops.[1] Only glucose tolerance tests were reported as having been used by alternative medical practitioners. Finally, five individuals obtained blood tests through private laboratories.

Further analysis of the information given suggested that, on the whole, clinical ecology methods were generally more oriented towards providing a basis for treatment than were conventional methods. In five cases, recipients of conventional allergy testing reported that their tests had been negative, so lacked implications for treatment. In several other cases, survey participants reported that they had been found, after skin tests, to be allergic to substances that did not appear to be causing their problems and that the cause of their symptoms remained undetected by these methods. One woman, for example, reported that the only allergy the tests had discerned was to a mould that grows on tomatoes. In three cases – two involving physical investigations and one involving allergy tests – people reported having been told that there was nothing the clinic or specialist could do to help them and in numerous other cases such an outcome was very strongly implied, since respondents reported that no help had in fact been offered after all the investigations had been completed.

By contrast, clinical ecology methods seemed to be geared towards treatment, which would either involve avoidance of the identified culprits or take the form of increasing the body's tolerance, by means of desensitizing drops or injections, or vitamin and mineral supplements. The experience of undergoing intensive and intrusive investigations on an in-patient basis for days or weeks at a time and having absolutely nothing to show for it was definitely not an outcome of clinical ecology investigations.

Another important difference that emerged from respondents' reports was that in their experience clinical ecology investigations were not fraught with adverse reactions when carried out under professional supervision. By contrast, survey participants reported at least four adverse reactions to substances used in conventional investigations. Two women described acute reactions to the 'fatty meal' mixture used to make the gall bladder contract during cholecystograms[2] and the mother of a little boy reported that on two occasions he had developed a rash on his scalp at the site where electrode paste had been applied during EEGs. In one case the rash had persisted for six months.

All in all, it seems reasonable to conclude from these findings that a proportion of conventional investigations are not of any immediate benefit to the allergic people who undergo them and that in some cases they are actually harmful. Professionally supervised clinical ecology investigations appeared to be generally more productive and without the risks associated with orthodox investigations. Alternative practitioners' investigative practices were not described in sufficient detail to make generalizations possible. However, a glucose tolerance test that is positive for reactive hypoglycaemia carries definite implications for treatment, so it may be the case that alternative investigations are also treatment-oriented.

Now let us consider, in turn, the main types of treatment which respondents obtained.

Conventional Medical Treatment

As might be predicted from the great variety of symptoms from which they suffered, survey respondents reported having had a great variety of treatments. Prescribed drugs and medicinal products comprised the largest category of treatments. These are shown in Table 21, with a breakdown of respondents' evaluations of their effectiveness.

One striking feature of the table is the dearth of strongly positive evaluations. Of a total of 113 prescriptions mentioned, only eight were reported to have been of great benefit, a rate of less than ten per cent. Second, the rate of adverse reactions reported is high — 15.04 per cent — roughly twice as high as the rate of greatly beneficial interventions. In particular, the pharmacological treatments listed under 'Other drugs' make a very poor showing. No respondents reported great benefit and

Table 21:   Evaluations of drugs and medicinal products received by survey respondents from conventional sources

Product or drug	Not evaluated	Little/no benefit	Some/ transient benefit	Moderate benefit	Great benefit	Adverse reaction
Antihistamines	4	1	–	–	1	–
Antihistamine Tablets	1	1	1	3	2	1
Antihistamine Inhalers	2	2	–	–	1	–
Nalcrom	2	–	1	2	–	2
Nosedrops/spray	–	1	–	1	–	1
Spirit lamp	1	–	–	–	–	–
Salves and creams	3	2	1	2	1	1
Analgesics	–	3	–	1	1	–
Migraine remedies	–	3	2	5	–	2
Tonic	1	–	–	–	–	–
Vitamin/mineral supplements	1	1	–	–	2	–
Psychotropic drugs	7	5	2	3	–	3
Bowel regulators	–	1	6	–	–	–
Steroids	1	–	1	2	–	1
Antibiotics	–	–	1	1	–	–
Other drugs	9	12	5	1	1	6

six, or nearly twenty five per cent, reported adverse reactions. Psychotropic drugs comprise the second largest category and the second leading cause of adverse reactions (17.65 per cent). If the entries in the moderate and great benefit columns are added together to represent the number of respondents reporting significant help from receiving the treatment, only six of the sixteen treatments are reported as having been of significant benefit by fifty per cent or more of the participants who reported having the treatment. Antihistamine tablets lead the field, with some 62.5 per cent reporting significant help. Vitamin and mineral supplements, migraine remedies, nosedrops and nasal sprays, steroids and antibiotics tie for second place, with fifty per cent of recipients reporting significant benefit. In one of the two cases where antibiotics were used, the condition in question was a complication of a respiratory allergy which the respondent said the doctor had refused to treat.

Taken as a whole, these findings suggest that, with an overall 'success rate' of 25.66 per cent (e.g. moderate and great benefit reported), conventional medical treatments leave something to be desired as an answer to the problems of many allergic people. This conclusion receives support from respondent's reports of their experience with other forms of medically prescribed treatments. These findings are shown in Table 22.

As in the previous table, very few significantly beneficial interventions are reported. However, since four of the thirty five interventions were said to have yielded great benefit, these non-medicinal interventions have around one and a half times the reported great benefit rate (11.43 per cent. vs. 8.62 per cent) of the drug interventions examined in the previous table. It is worth noting that the only intervention to be evaluated as greatly beneficial was advice on dietary avoidance. Thus doctors only reached fifty per cent success here when they gave advice that was characteristic of clinical ecology. But it should also be noted that the only adverse reaction reported in this table was to such advice. The respondent explained that the recommendation to avoid certain classes of food proved to be reasonably effective in preventing symptoms, but because no advice on rotating the remaining staples was given, further difficulties developed when the previously 'safe' foods were overused and tolerance of them was lost. Overall, only 17.14 per cent of the interventions included in this table were

Table 22:   Evaluations of other forms of conventional prescribed treatment

Treatment	Not evaluated	Little/no benefit	Some/ transient benefit	Moderate benefit	Great benefit	Adverse reaction
Surgical procedures (incl. ENT)	3	2	–	–	–	–
Rest	–	1	–	–	–	–
ECT	1	–	2	–	–	–
Slimming diet	–	1	–	–	–	–
Special foods on prescription	1	–	–	–	–	–
Advice on allergy	1	1	–	–	–	–
Advice on dietary avoidance	2	1	–	1	4	1
Group therapy	–	1	–	–	–	–
Speech therapy	–	1	–	–	–	–
Behaviour therapy	–	1	1	–	–	–
Relaxation therapy	–	–	–	1	–	–
Optician	–	1	–	–	–	–
'Treatment' unspecified	4	2	1	–	–	–

regarded by their recipients as having been significantly helpful. Because a high proportion were not evaluated, it remains possible that a greater number actually were beneficial, but at least the trend is consistent with the findings discussed earlier in the chapter.

If the figures from these two tables are combined to form global proportions of responses in each evaluative category, we find that 29.73 per cent of the medical interventions mentioned were not evaluated, 29.73 per cent were regarded as having been of little or no use, 16.22 per cent rated as having given only some or transient benefit, 15.54 per cent regarded as moderately helpful, and only 8.11 per cent seen as greatly beneficial. The overall 'success' rate, consisting of all responses in the moderate and great benefit categories, is 23.65 per cent and the rate of adverse reactions 12.16 per cent. Thus on the basis of the survey sample's reports, we reach the conclusion that doctors seem to have only about a one in four chance of providing their allergic patients with help that they report subsequently as having been significantly helpful; the chances of the patient being harmed by the intervention is of the order of one in eight. All in all, these findings do not yield a very encouraging picture of conventional approaches to the care of allergic people. Let us now see whether alternative medicine succeeds any better than the conventional offerings available within the NHS.

Alternative Medicine

In view of the poor performance of orthodox medical approaches to their problems, it is not surprising that many respondents turned to alternative medicine in the hope of finding solutions. How did they fare? The results of this analysis are presented in Table 23, with evaluations in the same categories as in the previous table.

The trend we see here is largely similar to what we saw for conventional medicine, but there are several important differences. Roughly the same proportion of interventions were not evaluated (29.73 per cent conventional, 27.78 per cent alternative), but there were many more reports of treatments that were of little or no benefit for alternative methods (29.73 per cent conventional, 44.44 per cent alternative) and also fewer of interventions that were of some or transient benefit (16.22 per cent conventional, 2.78 per cent alternative). The

Table 23:   Evaluations of alternative medical treatments

Treatment	Not evaluated	Little/no benefit	Some/ transient benefit	Moderate benefit	Great benefit	Adverse reaction
Acupuncture	1	5	–	–	1	–
Homoeopathy	4	3	1	1	–	1
Radionics	1	2	–	1	–	–
Psionic medicine with homoeopathy	–	–	–	–	1	–
Dowsing	1	–	–	1	–	–
Herbalist	1	–	–	–	–	–
Biofeedback	–	1	–	–	–	–
Naturopathy	–	1	–	1	–	–
Gerson therapy	–	–	–	–	1	–
Osteopath	–	1	–	–	–	–
Chiropractor	1	–	–	–	–	–
Faith healing	–	1	–	–	–	–
Spiritual healing	1	–	–	–	–	–
Hypnotherapy	–	1	–	–	–	–
Alternative medicine unspecified	–	–	–	–	1	–
Dietary advice	–	1	–	–	–	1

proportion of people reporting moderate benefit was marginally less for alternative medicine (15.54 per cent conventional, 11.11 per cent alternative). But a higher proportion reported great benefit than did so for conventional treatments (8.11 per cent conventional, 13.8 per cent alternative). The proportion of adverse reactions reported was less than half (5.55 per cent) for alternative medicine than for conventional (12.16 per cent). The overall success rate, as defined earlier, is slightly higher for alternative medicine (25.00 per cent) than for conventional (23.65 per cent). On the basis of these figures, it appears that, by and large, alternative medicine performs at about the same level as conventional medicine in the face of allergic suffering, which is to say, generally not very satisfactorily.

But this conclusion, which is based solely on quantitative comparisons, does not take the quality of benefit into account. If we compare respondents' reports of those alternative medical interventions that they found greatly beneficial with reports of the nature of the benefits received from conventional methods a rather different picture emerges. People who benefited from conventional methods mainly reported achieving good control over their symptoms, but, apart from those who were prescribed vitamins, they did not report either an increase in positive well-being or a permanent reduction in allergic sensitivity as a result of treatment. By contrast, several people who reported great benefit from alternative methods said that as a result of the treatment they no longer suffered from allergies. One woman whose otherwise unidentified alternative practitioner recommended a high protein, low carbohydrate diet for the control of hypoglycaemia said that since she adopted the diet she had never felt better. It appears, therefore, that the more holistic alternative interventions can result in a higher quality of improvement for certain sufferers than the mainly suppressive remedies of conventional allopathic medicine. It also appears that the outcome of alternative treatments are more clear-cut: either they work or they don't; the proportion of people who experience a degree of relief that falls short of appreciable or long-term significance is slight. But for the right people, alternative methods would appear to offer a dimension of effectiveness that is lacking in the orthodox approach based on drugs that suppress symptoms.

Having examined the performance of conventional and alternative medicine as evaluated by the survey respondents, let us now look at their assessments of the outcome of clinical ecology treatments.

Clinical Ecology

Participants's reports and evaluations of the clinical ecology treatments they underwent are shown in Table 24. The table includes all interventions carried out by or under the supervision of professionals indentifiable as practitioners of clinical ecology methods, whether or not they were actually members of the Society for Clinical Ecology. The main findings to emerge from these figures are that no one reported getting little or no benefit from clinical ecology treatments; that a high proportion reported great benefit; that when the overall 'success' rate is obtained, over half the reported interventions (54.05 per cent) are rated as having given moderate or great benefit, and that the rate of adverse reactions is even less than for alternative treatments. The overall impression derived from these results is that clinical ecology methods are quite clearly superior to both conventional and alternative methods in the rate at which those who undergo them report having been appreciably helped by their treatment.

As in the case of alternative medicine, the quality of benefit was often described in glowing terms. Hazel S, for example, an accountant in her mid-thirties, said that as a result of receiving private clinical ecology treatment for the past nineteen months, 'I am totally a new person. I no longer feel ill, always have lots of energy, my lack of confidence has gone and my nerves were never better. Life is worth living now, whereas before I could not bring myself to get up from the bed to face another day.' She rated the results of treatment as '100 per cent'. Others emphasized the improvements in what they were now able to accomplish in their lives. Nancy D, a residential child-care officer, described four years of fruitless GP treatment, a stint in psychiatic hospital, where she was given ECT, and finally, some seven years after her troubles had started, how she was sent to Dr Mackarness, then the country's only clinical ecologist, for investigation and treatment. Over the next eighteeen months she improved gradually and as of the time of her report had been well for six years. She reported that she was now able to hold down a fairly demanding job. Other reports of a similar nature were also given.

To facilitate a three-way comparison between the main

Table 24:   Evaluations of clinical ecology treatments

Treatment	Not evaluated	Little/no benefit	Some/ transient benefit	Moderate benefit	Great benefit	Adverse reaction
Elimination diet	–	–	–	3	10	1
Desensitization drops	3	–	5	1	1	–
Rotation	–	–	–	1	1	–
Desensitization injections	1	–	1	–	–	–
Urine therapy	1	–	–	–	–	–
Vaccine	1	–	1	–	–	1
Vitamin and mineral supplements	1	–	–	–	2	–
Fast	–	–	1	–	–	–
Clinical ecology unspecified	1	–	1	1	–	–

Table 25:   Comparison of evaluations of conventional medicine, alternative medicine, and clinical ecology treatments

Treatment	Not evaluated	Little/no benefit	Some/ transient benefit	Moderate benefit	Great benefit	Adverse reaction	'Success' (M and G)
Conventional	29.73	29.73	16.22	15.54	8.11	12.16	23.65
Alternative	27.78	44.44	2.78	11.11	13.89	5.55	25.00
Clinical ecology	21.62	—	23.32	16.22	37.83	5.41	54.05

approaches to treatment, the percentages of responses falling into each of the evaluative categories are given in Table 25. In view of these figures it seems fair to ask whether the apparently clear superiority of clinical ecology methods can be attributed to artefact. It would not appear to be accounted for by an appreciably lower rate of unevaluated responses. Another posibility is that the respondents who saw clinical ecologists were less seriously afflicted than those who didn't. But a separate analysis shows that the clinical ecology patients had both a higher average number of types of allergen than the sample as a whole (4.42 sample, 4.58 clinical ecology recipients) and a higher average number of symptoms (7.72 sample, 10.92 clinical ecology recipients). If these two figures are taken to represent a rough measure of the degree of affliction, it appears that clinical ecology outperforms the alternatives even with the 'handicap' of dealing with a more severely affected group of sufferers. At the same time it involves both less iatrogenic morbidity and less waste of resources in the form of interventions that do not help.

Nonetheless, clinical ecology also has its limitations. Respondents complained that it was difficult to come by clinical ecology services. When available privately, they were often impossibly costly to non-affluent sufferers. And in at least one case they had to be concealed from the respondent's general practitioner because he did not approve. The most obvious answer to these difficulties, of course would be to make clinical ecology clinics more widely available in the NHS than they are at the present time. But despite the advantages that would undoubtedly be gained by giving more people access to treatments that work better than conventional provisions, it seems sadly unlikely in the present economic climate that ecological facilities will be provided in the foreseeable future.

The results of our enquiry so far suggest what is likely to happen as a result: much avoidable suffering will continue, costly diagnostic and treatment resources will be wasted to no benefit, and people will continue to be lucky if their needs can be met by the public sector. Another outcome, which we will consider in more detail in the next chapter, is likely to be the proliferation of voluntary bodies to cater for the needs of sufferers. Finally, professionals other than doctors are likely to develop a certain expertise in advising people about home-based clinical ecology methods and people will turn to them for help if they cannot obtain it from their medical advisors. We shall consider this matter in the following section.

Other Sources of Help and Advice

Over a quarter of the sample reported seeking specific help and advice from those who were neither medical practitioners nor practitioners of alternative medicine but who might be expected to know something relevant to their difficulties. These sources of information and advice were generally mentioned without evaluation, though there were exceptions. The frequencies with which these informants were mentioned are shown in Table 26. Probably the main conclusion to be drawn from the variety of sources mentioned — which do not include contacts acquired through participation in self-help groups — is that allergic people are inclined to seek help and advice where they can find it: if they cannot obtain it from their doctors, they will try elsewhere. Indeed, as we shall see in the next chapter, the leading source of advice and support for survey participants was the many lay groups for sufferers that have come into existence in recent years to fill the great and unmet needs these people have for practical advice on living with their poorly understood condition.

Table 26:   Other sources of professional and practical help mentioned by respondents (excluding self-help groups)

Source	f
Clinical psychologist	6
Friends and fellow sufferers	3
Health visitor	2
Dietician	2
Food technologist	1
Psychiatric nurse	1
Biochemist	1
Natural food shop	1
Unspecified others	6

These findings lead to another conclusion, namely, that if full-scale medical clinical ecology services cannot be provided in the NHS for financial or other reasons, a less costly alternative might be to make more systematic use of interested paramedical personnel, such as clinical psychologists, health visitors, community nurses and dieticians. The case of Barbara G described earlier shows that non-medical therapists can successfully treat even quite complex cases of ecological disorder if allowed to do so. Thus if a proportion of paramedical staff in strategic positions were to become knowledgeable about environmental hypersensitivities and practical methods for their detection and management and were given scope to apply their knowledge, much of the reducible allergic suffering in the community might be attended to without recourse to more costly hospital-based medical facilities. Existing services could be used to back up the community-based practitioners and it would be anticipated that these services could be used more efficiently if the referrals were better focused, as they most likely would come from people who had an expert knowledge of the clinical phenomena of environmental hypersensitivity.

As we shall see in the following chapter, the majority of survey respondents used practical self-help methods to deal with their problems anyway and these methods compared favourably with the rest. The use of paramedical personnel with expertise in self-help methods would appear to have much to recommend it as a way of meeting many of the needs of allergy sufferers in the community. The potential benefits of this plan will become more evident in the following section which deals with one group of sufferers whose problems are especially poorly provided for – the parents of hyperactive children.

Experiences of Parents of Hyperactive Children Attempting to Find Help

As far as administrative provisions are concerned, hyperactive children do not exist. In the UK, children are classified as either 'maladjusted' or 'educationally subnormal (moderate)', but not as 'hyperactive'. Possibly for this reason, their parents find it difficult to obtain appropriate help through existing statutory channels, while medical services especially for such children are nonexistent. The mothers' reports have a depressing uniformity:

My oldest girl is hyperactive. The doctor kept telling me she would grow out of it. I was to give her sleeping draughts, which did not work; in fact they made her worse.

Vallergan and Phenergan were prescribed two or three times a week to get some sleep. Although the doctor said the baby was hyperactive there was nothing else they could do.

When he was an infant the GP prescribed various sleeping medicines but nothing worked. At age two and a half a GP refused to prescribe sleeping medicine and a doctor was never consulted again about hyperactivity. No investigations were ever carried out regarding the sleeplessness or hyperactivity.

We haven't sought medical attention for hyperactivity. Speech therapy for stammer was not successful (no apparent physical cause and the therapist said he would probably grow out of it).

. . . I consulted our GP after a very long (two months) bout of bad eyes. Having already seen an optician three times in eighteen months and having been told there was nothing wrong with my son's vision, I asked GP for skin tests. All came up negative. Then I asked to be referred to a paediatrician. By the time my appointment came up (a wait of three months) I'd learned a great deal about my son's food allergies from pulse tests. When we eventually saw the paediatrician, he confessed we knew more about the problems than he did. He hadn't before considered food allergy causing hyperactivity.

The mothers' reports of treatments and advice obtained were somewhat more varied. One hyperactive child was fortunate to obtain an effective rotation diet from a clinical ecologist. Another was treated by her mother, a former SRN, with a diet worked out by means of pulse testing. Another mother, who was given a copy of Coca's book, *The Pulse Test*,[3] and general instructions for use by a psychiatric nurse, managed to do the same for her child. But the main source of effective outside help for these families was the self-help and special-interest groups to which they belonged — the Hyperactive Children's Support Group, Action Against Allergy, local allergy groups, and Sanity.

If lay groups can successfully provide vital information, advice and support to the families of these children, it seems unlikely that at least some of the professionals such as health visitors, educational and clinical psychologists, nursery nurses and others who come into contact with the children would be unable to acquire some of the necessary knowledge and expertise. Especially if doctors are unable or unwilling to do so, it would make enormous sense to inculcate the knowledge in other professionals at many different places in the system of care provision. Not all of these 'grassroots experts' would necessarily need to take on cases for 'treatment'; it would probably suffice, in most cases, simply to transmit to those who required it the information necessary for them to undertake dietary investigation and remediation on their own. Parents have certainly shown themselves capable of implementing these diagnostic and treatment strategies on their own without benefit of professional advice and support, but it would probably reduce the strain on them to obtain such advice when the need for it first arose, in a systematic and planned way, rather than several years later after just happening to come across a magazine article or a media programme on the topic.

Meanwhile, the unmet needs continue to mount up and the impetus to involve professionals, so far, is coming from the lay groups themselves rather than from the professions. The children continue to float about in administrative limbo.[4] Their numbers increase as the many forms of environmental pollution that interact in disrupting the function of their developing brains proliferate. Public-health spending diminishes, so that services become progressively less likely to be provided. Making use of existing professional resources to disseminate information that could enable the families of hyperactive children to help themselves would contribute towards alleviating a severe and growing social problem.

Some might object that this plan accepts the status quo, the polluted environment, the resistance of doctors to the idea that environmental factors can have adverse effects on children's behaviour, the food-labelling legislation that allows manufacturers to conceal the ingredients of food products from the consumer, and so forth, and that it might be more effective in the long run to clean up the environment, promote research that will convince the doctors, change food-labelling regulations, and the like. The objection is certainly valid but overlooks the legitimacy of the needs of children and families who are suffering now. Scouring the environment of all the unnatural and toxic factors that are rampant in the post-technological era would require a long time and a lot of social action, financial resources, and other rare facilities, and meanwhile many people would continue to suffer the consequences of exposure to the unscoured mess. Are they to be considered expendable? And, if so, who is going to take the decision?

Second, the objection assumes that short-term first aid and long-term preventive measures are somehow necessarily mutually exclusive. This assumption is certainly unnecessary. There is no fundamental conflict of interests between trying to do something for people who are suffering now and trying to do something to prevent others from suffering later. In fact, help for present-day sufferers might facilitate long-term environmental clear-up by releasing funds, which would otherwise be used to no good purpose in perseverative efforts to deal with the problem by denying that it exists. All the fruitless sleeping draughts, medical consultations, speech-therapy sessions, optician appointments etc. are costing the taxpayer money that might more profitably be expended elsewhere. If national spending on health is likely to decrease, it becomes all the more imperative that we make more efficient use of our resources. The lay groups have provided an evidently workable model of a grassroots solution to some of the problems of childhood hyperactivity, in the short term at least (it is too early to tell about the long term); my suggestion is that this model be adapted for use by certain strategically placed professionals, so that in ten years' time, when the numbers of hyperactive children can be predicted to have soared, the parents of these unfortunate young environmental casualties are spared some of the frustration, aggravation, and waste that the present generation of parents have encountered in their attempts to obtain help within the system.

The situation of parents of hyperactive children highlights the key role that lay self-help groups for sufferers can play in the management of complex environmental hypersensitivities in Britain today. In the following chapter, we shall examine respondents' participation in these groups in more detail.

6.

Self-Help

In the absence of much effective outside help, respondents were largely thrown back upon their own resources. They were asked to describe their self-help efforts to deal with their condition as follows:

> What have you done about the problems on your own initiative, without outside help? In particular, have you read anything about them, kept diet records or recorded symptoms, or tried elimination dieting, or any other experiments with food or chemical exposure? Have you tried any self-prescribed remedies you may have heard or read about or worked out for yourself? Have these efforts been a help?

In this chapter we shall look at respondents' answers to this question. The analysis is based on the replies of the eighty four respondents who answered the question. One, for some unknown reason, left the whole page of the questionnaire blank. But all the rest describe some form of self-help activity.

The results of the analysis of their responses are shown in Table 27. The outstanding features of the table are the wide range of self-help methods reported, the large number of reports (a total of 367 items mentioned) and the high proportion that were reported to be either moderately or greatly beneficial. Of the seventeen types of activity reported, only two, food testing

Table 27:   Self-help activities as evaluated by respondents (n = 84)

Activity	Not evaluated	Little/no benefit	Some/ transient benefit	Moderate benefit	Great benefit	Adverse reaction
Elimination diet and avoidance						
of offending foods	5	–	3	37	34	–
Diet/symptom records	5	–	–	2	19	–
Pulse test	3	–	–	1	7	–
Self-monitoring	–	–	–	2	3	–
Food testing	5	2	–	–	4	6
Reading	11	–	–	26	36	–
Self-help groups/special interest						
organizations	3	–	–	6	25	–
Avoidance of physical						
precipitants	19	–	2	20	16	–
Self-prescribed remedies	7	3	1	5	5	1
Self-prescribed vitamins	1	–	1	2	8	–8
Other information-seeking	5	–	–	1	11	–
Rotation diet	–	1	–	–	3	–
Private blood tests	1	–	–	4	–	–
Pure and simple foods	–	–	–	–	6	–
Fasting	–	–	–	–	1	–
Meditation	–	–	–	1	–	–
Conferences	1	–	–	1	1	–

(36.36 per cent) and self-prescribed remedies (47.62 per cent) were reported to have been significantly helpful in less than fifty per cent of cases mentioned. Both of these figures are nonetheless considerably higher than the overall averages for conventional and alternative medicine. The effectiveness of self-prescribed remedies, as assessed by respondents, also seems to be appreciably higher than that of the majority of medically-prescribed remedies reported in the previous chapter.

From these findings it seems reasonable to conclude that allergic people tend to be extremely active in the self-management of their condition and that their efforts compare quite favourably in outcome with those of the professionals from whom they reported having sought help.

The relative ineffectiveness of food testing as a self-help measure seems to derive from a number of sources. In two cases it was reported to be inconclusive, largely because of the individuals' inability to limit concurrent exposure to physical allergens, reactions to which obscured the effects of test reintroductions of foods. The figures were also lowered by the relatively high proportion of unevaluated responses. The high proportion of adverse reactions reported is perhaps only to be expected, since the purpose of food testing is to determine the safety or otherwise of the test food precisely by seeing if it provokes an adverse reaction. If these inevitable adverse effects are excluded from a calculation of the percentage of self-help interventions that were reported to have lead to adverse reactions, leaving the proportion of reactions that might be regarded as unanticipated, the figure falls to less than half of one percent (.48 percent). But even if they are included, the proportion of interventions producing morbidity is still considerably lower than those reported for any of the types of professional treatment that we examined in the previous chapter. The remaining adverse reaction was reported by a respondent who became hypersensitive to sodium bicarbonate through using it too frequently in self-treating his reactions to other substances.[1]

Thus it seems that the worst the overwhelming majority of self-help interventions can do is fail to work; they are very unlikely to damage their practitioners. And by respondents' own reports, their own efforts seem more likely than not to be helpful.

We may now compare the overall results for the four types of

Table 28:   Comparative effectiveness of conventional, alternative medicine, clinical ecology and self-help as evaluated by survey participants

Type of treatment	Not evaluated	Little/no benefit	Some/ transient benefit	Moderate benefit	Great benefit	Adverse reaction	M and G
Conventional	29.73	29.73	16.22	15.34	8.11	12.16	23.65
Alternative	27.78	44.44	2.78	11.11	13.89	5.55	25.00
Clinical ecology	21.62	—	24.32	16.22	37.83	5.41	54.05
Self-help	17.98	1.63	2.18	29.43	48.77	2.18	78.20

treatment: conventional and alternative medicine, clinical ecology and self-help. The respective proportions of reports falling into each of the evaluative categories for the four approaches are shown in Table 28. It appears that respondents tended to evaluate their self-help efforts more often than the other forms of help they received. In at least three quarters of cases they reported their own activities to have yielded significant benefit. On respondents' own subjective criteria, self-help seems clearly superior to the other types of help that they tried.

The figure of 78.2 percent of interventions being reported as helpful is consistent with previous findings in the area of self-help. A study of people's self-help behaviour in depression, carried out in the early 1970s in London, found respondents reporting that an average of 71.99 percent of their antidepressive activities were either moderately or very helpful, by means of ratings on a 3-point scale.[2] The similarity of the two figures suggests that people may generally find about three quarters of their self-help efforts to be helpful.

This possibility raises an interesting question, namely, why people's own efforts, which normally involve so much less technology than even the most basic hospital investigations, should seem to be so much more effective than the best that professionals appear to be able to offer for these conditions. And why do people's self-help efforts apparently result in a much lower proportion of adverse reactions? Although objective answers to these questions cannot be given, there seems to be a number of factors which, taken collectively, go far towards explaining the results.

First, sufferers, who are often acutely and uncomfortably aware of the fact that they have a problem do not resort to dismissing its existence or to trivializing its importance by writing it off as due to their 'nerves', their 'age', or to 'thinking about their troubles too much', or to construing it as something their child will 'grow out of'. All these typical brush-offs were reported to have come from doctors or other professionals by survey respondents. The following excerpts from the questionnaires refer to such brush-off situations:

I was thought to be suffering from 'nerves' and 'anxiety'. Tranquillizers were prescribed for a while until I refused to take them. (Woman, aged fifty)

My doctor said that the headaches and migraines were due to stress and nerves. (Woman, aged fifty-nine)

No treatment at all — until three years ago I was told that it was nerves. (Woman, ages fifty-six)

In the past, other GPs told me my symptoms were due to 'nerves', to 'being too introspective' and suchlike. I once asked one to explain to me how 'being too introspective' could produce the symptoms. He had no explanation, of course. I think he was really just trying to get rid of me. (Woman, aged thirty-five)

My doctor's opinion is that if I stop thinking about my troubles they will disappear. . . My reply was that I refused to give up the fight and would seek other help. (Woman, aged fifty-eight)

Most [doctors] seem to think it is all in the mind and is a way of craving for attention. . . It was when I started working in a medical library that I found out that my doctor had 'fobbed me off'. (Woman, aged twenty-four)

The situation seems to be much the same if the patient is a child about whom the mother is seeking advice:

He [GP] wouldn't listen to me when I tried to tell him what my daughter was like but insisted on giving me tranquillizers, which I threw away. (Mother of a twelve year-old girl)

I consulted medical friends in the past who laughed and stated it was 'in the mind'. . .I took my children to [a specialist children's hospital] and was told that there were some children like mine and they would probably grow out of it. (Mother of two adult children, both allergic)

There always seemed to be something wrong with her. She was continually suffering from headaches, tummy-aches, colds, sore throats, fleeting itchy rashes and various other aches and pains. I was constantly taking her along to the doctor's surgery but my doctor could never find anything wrong with her and insisted that she was a very healthy child. (Mother of a twelve year-old girl)

I took him to the doctor many times as he was always so tired and complaining of backache and very tearful. Various tests were carried out but we were eventually told there was nothing wrong and if it continued he would have to see a psychiatrist. (Mother of a fifteen year-old boy)

Where medical advisers display a tendency to dismiss or minimize problems which sufferers present to them for solution, sufferers themselves start from the premise that they have got a problem and that labelling and homilies won't make it disappear. Acknowledgement of the existence of the problem, while it does not in itself entail a solution, is obviously essential as a first step. The fact that sufferers take this step undoubtedly contributes substantially to their greater success in finding solutions than many of their medical advisors can claim.

Second, because sufferers have got to live with the problem day in and day out until a solution is found, they are highly motivated to find a satisfactory outcome. The same motivation to succeed cannot necessarily be assumed to exist in the doctors to whom these patients turn for help. Part of the difficulty here is situational: some doctors, particularly those at hospital-based clinics, may see a given patient on only one or two occasions and are likely to conceive of their role in a narrow and technological way – possibly taking a history, sending the sufferer for routine tests and, if nothing obvious turns up, either sending him or her back to the GP or on to another specialist. Apart from the GP, it seems rare for anyone professionally involved to be expected to take responsibility for seeing that a solution is not only sought but found. The respondents' reports of their encounters with their GPs suggest that while this may happen in rare instances, it is exceptionally uncommon. One woman, who reported that by badgering her GP until he was so fed up with her that he sent her to hospital, where she succeeded in obtaining some treatment, said that until she was twenty-one her doctor thought she was exaggerating the problem – a very violent hypersensitivity to even trace amounts of egg. 'He told me that there was very little that could be done anyway and he *didn't* recommend any kind of treatment. He said it would interfere with schooling, etc. In other words, he wasn't interested at all.' This sort of report was considerably more common than that of the woman who said that her GP had diagnosed her condition as allergic, sent to her to several leading specialists, treats her with every respect and tries to help in every way he can. Respondents undoubtedly obtained better results from their own efforts than most of their doctors because they tried harder to find solutions to their problems.

Third, sufferers do better by their own efforts because they bring to their attempts an attitude that we might call *ecological realism*. Sufferers know what is and what is not feasible within the limits of their own particular social, psychological, economic and physical niches, and what their resources can and cannot bear. Their practical, concrete awareness of the context into which interventions are, willy-nilly, going to have to fit makes it unlikely that they will resort to formulating idealistic 'solutions' which in sheer practical terms are totally unfeasible. Many respondents reported having been given suggestions and advice to follow that might have made sense in an ideal world but which are absolutely senseless in terms of what was realistically possible for them. The most glaring example of completely impractical advice was one woman's report that a doctor had advised her to 'go live on top of an Alp' as a means of controlling her respiratory difficulties. Another woman reported that she had been unable to follow the dietary advice she had been given because she simply could not afford the costly high-protein foods recommended. She was raising four children as a single parent, with only basic Social Security income. By contrast to advice that is impossible to follow, sufferers will come up with plans that they can actually implement and the relevance of their plans to their actual circumstances is another factor that contributes to the greater success of their efforts.

Fourth, sufferers would seem to succeed better than the experts because they are more likely to persist in their efforts to find a satisfactory solution. From many respondents' reports of their medical encounters, it seemed that often the doctor's underlying strategy might be phrased, 'Maybe try something and if that doesn't work tell the patient nothing can be done.' One fifty-seven year-old housewife described the medical help she had received as 'a fatalistic shrug by the GPs, even though Dixarit tried for some years did not help'. Several respondents said that after hospital investigations had been completed, they were dismissed without treatment or constructive advice. A forty-six year-old woman wrote as follows: 'The hospital confirmed after tests and a biopsy that I was allergic to certain foods which had caused my small intestine to be damaged but could offer no further help. They said that with care I would survive.' A fifty-four year-old man told a similar story: 'The specialist was sympathetic and after routine tests explained that there were many things about the digestive system that were not fully understood; I would have to learn to live with my condition.' He carried on searching and eventually found help from another source. By contrast to this sort of medical abdication of responsibility for seeing that help sought becomes help actually obtained, the sufferer's motto most often seems to be, 'Try something and if that doesn't help keep trying till you find something that does.' Sufferers' greater persistence in the face of unsuccessful initial interventions undoubtedly contributes substantially to their higher success rate.

Fifth, the tendency to persist longer in the search for an effective solution entails both a greater openness to alternative possibilities and a greater awareness of what the available options are. Because many allergic people read so widely on the topics of allergy, clinical ecology, alternative medicine, and nutrition, they are as a whole probably much more knowlegeable about these matters than many of their medical advisors – a fact which some of their doctors were reported to have acknowledged. Because they seek information from a wider range of sources, sufferers raise the likelihood that they will encounter a solution to their own particular problem, if one exists. But they are not only exposed to a wider range of options; they are also, as a group, much more receptive to new ideas than their conservatively-trained medical advisers. The difference in attitude is terribly important. Being fundamentally pragmatic in outlook, sufferers are less likely than professionals to dismiss new ideas out of hand if these ideas do not happen to conform to contemporary conventional wisdom about allergy or if they reliably lead to results, the mechanism of which remains unknown. Sufferers would rather get better on unscientific grounds than continue to suffer on scientific ones. This is not to say that they are uncritical; rather, they use different criteria than doctors to assess new approaches. They are more interested in finding out whether the method has been found to help in cases like theirs than in whether it was found in double-blind, randomized, controlled trials to outperform some drug or other. As long as the proposed new method is reasonably safe, reasonably inexpensive, and under their own control to obtain and test, many sufferers are willing to have a go at just about anything. If they have their own doubts, they can be ingenious at devising tests to allay them. Thus the two respondents who reported having tried a pendulum both told of having conducted their own tests. The first, a housewife of sixty-one, wrote: 'On a friend's recommendation I have used a pendulum to discover whether or not a food is safe and in spite of my doubts this is reasonably accurate, even on blind tests.' The other, a forty-nine year-old clerk-typist, gave a more detailed description:

> I have. . . tried. . . (as a matter of interest and making no claims for it) the pendulum. A bit of a party trick, really, but it is remarkably consistent. I once put drinking water in a cup and water from the hot tap into an identical cup, then covered both and my son changed them around. I didn't look but *every* time I was able to tell which was which.

From these reports it seems as though sufferers ask themselves, 'What have I got to lose?' and if the odds appear favourable, they get on and try it.

Sixth, in addition to requiring much less 'scientific proof' than doctors before being willing to try a new approach, sufferers also seem to differ from the experts in the goals at which they aim many of their interventions. From their reports of their medical encounters, it seemed that the goal of most medical interventions in these people's problems was the alleviation of symptoms rather than the discovery of causes – either immediate or long-range. Some respondents reported that they were given symptomatic treatment without benefit of any investigations. Other reported that when a few routine tests failed to reveal obvious pathology, they were also given either symptomatic treatment or, in some cases, none at all. The following reports show a depressing stereotypy:

> No investigations were ever carried out regarding the sleeplessness or hyperactivity. (Mother of an eight year-old boy)

> No GP helped me in any way other than by tranquillizers or antidepressants. My psychiatrist was supportive but could only offer medication. No investigation into what was

causing the depression was done. (Housewife and mother, aged fifty-three)

Nobody could find the cause of my abdominal pain until we met Dr Mackarness. I have had many drugs given to me which made me feel much worse. I improved soon by going on the elimination diet. (Secretary, aged twenty-three)

Only investigations – eye examinations at hospital and blood test. . . Medication prescribed often seemed to make sickness much worse and did not relieve pain. Needed to take more and more drugs until diet eliminated the needs for all drugs. (Teacher, aged forty-seven)

Thorough gastro-enterological investigation at hospital (barium follow-through, gall bladder X-rays, jejunal biopsy). No treatment; nothing found to be wrong). (Housewife, aged forty-four)

Initially I had wide investigations, ECG, blood tests, urine tests, X-rays, etc. Apart from a slight urinary tract infection no abnormalities could be found. Later I was prescribed Sectral to control the rapid pulse. This was only effective for four months until further foods caused the rapid pulse rate even with the tablets. (Housewife, aged sixty-one)

I have had thyroid tests, IVP, etc. I have had every drug in the psychiatric book but without success. (Nurse, aged thirty-three)

These reports characterize the typical medical approach to these people's perplexing problems.

Although some respondents (chiefly those for whom it was effective) appeared to be content with symptomatic relief, others clearly felt that more was needed. Many wanted to know what was making them ill, so that they could do something about avoiding exposure to it. A housewife of thirty-four, mother of four affected children, stated her position as follows: 'It's better to eat the correct foods than to live on antihistamines, which may have bad side effects.' Another woman echoed her view and amplified it:

I'd rather go to some lengths to avoid exposure to the things that make me feel so ill than resort to taking drugs to suppress the symptoms of my failure to do so. You can never tell what the long-term effect of repeated allergic reactions on the body's tolerance will be and I would rather not have to find out the hard way.

She introduced another theme which several other respondents also stressed:

> . . .Ideally, of course, it should be possible to alter the body's tolerance so that allergic reactions no longer happen. I'm still looking into ways of doing that.

This theme recurs in the protocols from several others. One young woman reported that although an elimination diet had been quite successful in preventing her disabling symptoms, she was nonetheless about to start a course of homoeopathy 'to remove the cause' of her allergic reactivity. Her sentiment was echoed by a housewife of sixty-three:

> . . .I feel there is a deeper cause – one which causes the allergy. It is unnatural to be allergic to good and wholesome foods such as wheat, eggs, milk etc. We should research into what causes allergies in the first place rather than what effects the allergens have. We are still only treating symptoms.

Two other women reported that as a result of treatment which removed the causes of their allergic tendency, they no longer suffered from allergies. Both of these were treatments obtained by exploring the world of alternative medicine. From these reports there is a suggestion that many sufferers aim higher than doctors in the goals they set for themselves. Many want life to be more than a perpetual popping of pills between laps of the obstacle course. The fact that they aim higher undoubtedly contributes greatly to their higher achievements in finding relief.

How do we explain the lower proportion of adverse reactions incurred by sufferers undergoing self-treatment than amongst the same sufferers undergoing medical treatment? One obvious reason is that lay people haven't got access to as many potentially dangerous drugs as doctors do. But another reason is that they probably apply a different criterion of acceptable risk in weighing up the potential hazards versus the potential benefits involved in procedures and remedies than their doctors. And, being more aware of their own idiosyncratic susceptibilities, they are more acutely conscious than doctors of where hidden risks might be lurking. On the whole, doctors appear to assess risks with reference to some hypothetical 'average person' (who almost by definition is not allergic to common substances), whereas sufferers evaluate risks in relation to their own unique personal hypersensitivites. As a result, they are much less likely to expose themselves to medicinal substances that could prove to be allergenic.

Another difference relevant here is that sufferers are in a much better position than doctors to notice the beginnings of an adverse reaction to any intervention: they get the unwelcome information immediately, whereas the doctor may not hear of it, if at all, until days or weeks later. Because they are the ones who have to suffer the consequences and are thus in a position to know that consequences are being suffered, they are less likely than doctors to perseverate for long with remedies they find harmful. Moreover, if they get symptoms that begin when they start the remedy and stop when they discontinue it, they are likely to be able to draw the obvious conclusion. A number of sufferers described being told categorically that the drugs they were being given could not possibly have produced the side effects they reported. Because they are in a position to demonstrate the contrary to their own satisfaction, sufferers know better and can act accordingly.

Finally, another difference that helps to account for the lower rate of adverse reactions reported as resulting from self-help measures is that many of the self-help tactics adopted by sufferers do not take the form of self-treatment, but are, rather, educational in nature, so cannot be said to carry risks of adverse reactions in the usual sense. Such activities – attending meetings of self-help groups, writing to manufacturers for information, replacing allergenic household equipment with hypoallergenic materials, and the like – are free of the sorts of risks intrinsic in introducing chemicals into the body or undergoing invasive investigation procedures in hospital. Since a large proportion of the self-help activities reported were of these risk-free types, the finding that self-help caused fewer adverse reactions is only what would be expected.

Since reading and participation in self-help groups were so often mentioned, it will be useful to look at them in more detail.

Table 29:   Reading reported by survey sample

(a) Titles and authors	f	(b) Other authors	f	(c) Other reading	f
Mackarness *Not All in the Mind*	32	Randolph	4	Books unspecified	14
Coca *The Pulse Test*	7	Rowe	2	Reading unspecified	12
Feingold *Why Your Child is*		Taube	2	Popular media	8
Hyperactive	6	Mandell	1	Anything–everything	5
Dickey *Clinical Ecology*	4	Rinkel	1	Articles	4
Mackarness *Chemical Victims*	2	Rea	1	Medical textbooks	3
Williams *Nutrition Against Disease*	2	Forman	1	Hospital information sheet on	
Crook *Can Your Child Read?*		Eagle	1	dust allergy	1
Is He Hyperactive?	1	Pfeiffer	1	Elimination diet plan	1
Forsythe *Asthma, Hay Fever and*		Fredericks and Goodman	1	*Here's Health*	1
Other Allergies	1	Richet *et al*	1	Reading strongly implied	15
Dufty *Sugar Blues*	1	Yudkin	1		
Price *Nutrition and Physical*		Sneddon	1		
Degeneration	1				
Moyle *Asthma and Hay Fever*	1				
Crook *Are You Allergic?*	1				

Reading

Reading about allergy and related topics was mentioned or strongly implied by eighty-seven percent of the group. The reading matter reported is shown in Table 29. The respondents' reports are given in three sections: (a) titles and authors; (b) authors only; (c) other. The range of reading that respondents actually did was undoubtedly much larger than the books and authors specifically mentioned by name, since some reported reading 'widely', 'anything' and 'everything I can get hold of on the subject of allergies'.

Mackarness lead the feld with *Not All in the Mind,* which was mentioned by 37.65 percent of the sample. This finding highlights the key role this book has played in raising British consciousness of masked allergy and clinical ecology. The fact that *Chemical Victims* was not so widely reported is due to the fact that the book first appeared in March 1980, after most of the questionnaire had already been returned. Clinical ecology publications, some of them quite technical, were generally the most frequently reported (Mackarness, Coca, Dickey, Crook, Randolph, Rowe, Taube, Mandell, Rinkel, Rea, Forman, and Richet *et al* – this latter evidently read in the Rowe translation of 1930). Orthomolecular works, books on hyperactivity, hypoglycaemia, diet, nutrition, vitamins, alternative medicine, and medical tests were also reported.

Books were often mentioned by name in the context of the respondent's discovery of a way of conceptualizing his or her previously intractable problem in a way that made it, in principle, soluble. From their accounts we hear not only what they read but how they applied what they had learnt from their reading when trying to solve their problems.

Doris J, a forty-nine year-old housewife living in the Midlands, tells a typical story. She wrote that although she could 'write a book on the subject' of the medical attention she sought for her headaches and migraines, the drugs she received in their numbers 'had no real effect'. Then she joined Action Against Allergy and was sent a copy of Mackarness's *Not All in the Mind.* On the basis of her reading, she started to keep diet records and tried elimination dieting, with the result that she was able to identify fifteen environmental precipitants of her headaches, which she now can avoid. Although she still gets the odd headache from time to time, her formerly severe and incapacitating migraines had been a thing of the past for nearly three years at the time of her report. 'Basically my husband and I have worked this out for ourselves from reading Dr Mackarness's book,' she wrote and acknowledged her gratitude to Mrs Nathan Hill of Action Against Allergy for having put her on the right track by sending her the book.

Andrew F, a fifty-two year old administrator, suffers from painful blisters on the edges of his hands and feet. His report is similar to Doris's:

> My physician tried creams, which made no difference; so he sent me to the hospital dermatology department. I was given all the standard tests and was found to be allergic to house dust and to cats, but no cause [for the blisters] could be found. I followed Richard Mackarness's plan of going off each substance in my diet for five days at a time, and at last found that white bread gave me a severe reaction (enough to bring a crop of blisters for biopsy when the consultant asked me to cause some)

A similar story comes from others.

Ruth M, the mother of a six year-old hyperactive boy, said that she was given Coca's book *The Pulse Test*, by a psychiatric nurse, together with 'a rough outline of what to do':

> I tried this on my son and in four weeks concluded he was allergic to grain and I subsequently eliminated this from his diet. In about ten weeks after that it became apparent that dairy products and various other foods were 'wrong'. Since eliminating all these, my son is a very much calmer child, concentrates well and sits still without fidgeting. His pulse remains in the 60's range and only rises into the 70's after infractions. Before the elimination diet his pulses were very high – 90's and 100's.

Ruth's story is echoed by Betty C, whose hyperactive son is a few years older. She said she read Crook's *Can Your Child Read? Is He Hyperactive?*[3] and 'eliminated white flour, white sugar and milk from his diet and continued to monitor food and effect and eliminated suspect or obvious foods affecting him'. The result was equally good.

Dierdre E, a middle-aged housewife who suffered from intractable migraines and colitis, wrote:

Read *Not All in the Mind*. Decided I felt as though there was poison in my blood. It had to be something I did every day to have so many bad effects. With always being so sick I was very underweight so ate fattening foods. Drank pints of milk. Decided to go on a low-fat diet. Diet of great help. Colitis cleared up completely. Migraine less severe, less frequent.

Hilary O, a twenty-nine year-old lecturer who gets itchy rashes, depression, and a painfully bloated abdomen which has undergone medical investigations to no avail, reported:

Having read Mackarness's book *Not All in the Mind*, I experimented with diet for a while. Felt considerably better both mentally and physically during the period I was being 'strong minded' and sticking to foods considered safe in Mackarness's terms.

Megan T, a nurse, said that she did not find the elimination diet she undertook initially in order to work out why she always felt unwell to be personally effective because she only developed delayed reactions to her allergens:

Eventually I came across Dr A. Coca's book *The Pulse Test* and by keeping pulse records was eventually able to pinpoint the offending foods with success.

'I have ready anything that comes my way regarding allergies,' she added.

These accounts are typical of many others given by survey participants and illustrate the group's tendency to try out the ideas encountered in reading in their attempts to sort themselves out when medical help has proved unavailable or unavailing.

Self-help Groups

In their analysis of the characteristic types of problems for which self-help groups come into existence, Robinson and Henry[4] differentiate between 'normal' and 'abnormal' problems. Briefly, 'normal' problems are those which can be dealt with by conventional problem-solving methods or else conveniently swept under the carpet. 'Abnormal' problems, by contrast, have three common features: first, they are indefinable or not identifiable as problems and are thus not readily diagnosed; second, if they are diagnosed, it is as incurable – the experts cannot paper over them and have them quietly disappear; and third, the conventional way of handling them causes distress. Moreover, the fact that sufferers do not oblige by getting better, shutting up, or vanishing, leads others to regard *them* as problems and to deal with them by adopting a stigmatizing attitude. As we have seen so far, the problems of many allergic people display the three prime features of 'abnormal' problems. And as we shall see in the chapter on social reactions, they also entail the stigmatization of sufferers.

Against this background it would be predicted that food allergy and chemical hypersensitivity would provide a nexus for the existence of self-help groups and the prediction is amply borne out by our respondents' reports.

In their efforts to find relief from their hypersensitivities and symptoms, respondents received much help from self-help groups and voluntary organizations for sufferers and others with this particular interest. Two reported having founded such groups themselves in order to pass on to others in similar circumstances the support and advice they might need while sorting out their difficulties and living with the resultant solution. The organizations mentioned are shown in Table 30.

Table 30:   Groups mentioned by respondents (n = 33)

Group	f
Action Against Allergy	10
Hyperactive Children's Support Group	6
Food Allergy Association	5
Food Allergy Club	4
Sanity	4
Chemical Victims	3
Schizophrenia Association of Great Britain	3
Feingold Association of America	3
British Migraine Association	2
McCarrison Society	1

The figures add up to a higher total than the figure given in Table 27 because a number of respondents mentioned more than one group or organization.

What sufferers gained from their contact with these groups can be gleaned from a selection of their reports. Information and advice were prominent themes. The mother of one hyperactive boy reported that she had tried an additive-free diet on her own but 'made many mistakes'. Then she joined the Hyperactive Children's Support Group and followed their diet and advice: 'result – good'. Another mother reported 'the Hyperactive Children's Support Group has been very helpful; the foods on their "banned" list have bad results' on her children.

Information about relevant practitioners was another offering of some of the groups. A middle-aged housewife reported: 'I joined a group that meets monthly who put me in touch with an allergy doctor and he is still treating me. At last I feel I am getting somewhere.' Other respondents reported having been referred to clinical ecologists through Action Against Allergy. Certain services, such as private blood tests, were also available through Sanity, and another respondent spoke of intending to obtain a hair test for trace minerals through the auspices of the Hyperactive Children's Support Group.

Moral support and encouragement were commonly reported to have been found through groups. Jennifer H, a sixty-one year-old housewife, wrote: 'I joined the Food Allergy Association. I cannot stress too highly the help and support I have obtained from this group, meeting fellow sufferers, sharing hints, and hearing speakers on allergy and related subjects.' Brian G, whom we heard from earlier, wrote that he had been trying elimination diets inconclusively on his own, with interesting but frustrating results: 'It was at this stage when despair was setting in that I was referred to AAA. I read *Not All in the Mind* by Dr Mackarness, which encouraged me to keep trying.' Through AAA he was also referred to the ecology clinic where, under expert guidance, he feels he is now 'making considerable progress'. Betty S, a middle-aged teacher, is a member of Dr Mackarness's Chemical Victims Club. Her comment: 'Advice and encouragement much appreciated'. Through participation in the club, Betty has read books on food allergy and now spreads the word herself: 'I tell people who seem to be suffering from similar complaints; particularly those told by doctors that "their age" is the trouble.' Nancy D, another member of the same club, writes of her experience: 'This gave me the opportunity to talk to other allergic people initially and also gave me a great deal of support in dealing with my problems. I still attend regularly as I still need the contact of other sufferers.' Helen F, a housewife of fifty-seven, wrote in a similar vein of a different organization: 'I joined the British Migraine Association twelve years ago and it did my morale a lot of good and enabled me to speak of my troubles to my family and others.' And Alice A, a fifty-two year-old housewife, who only joined the Food Allergy Association after her own dietary problems had been sorted out, noted that '. . .however, there always seems to be more to learn and I can help others by my experience'. She now introduces to the group some of the people she meets who have similar problems and adds that, 'The number I hear of is steadily growing.'

Other members of these groups, notably AAA, emphasized the value of the books they had been sent, lent, or directed towards. Marge E wrote: 'I have read many books supplied to me through the kindness of Mrs A. Nathan Hill. I have found these most helpful.' And Doris J, whose story we have heard, wrote: 'I was greatly helped in my search by Mrs Nathan Hill, who sent me Dr Mackarness's book.' Others also gave similar reports.

We can now summarise what the groups offer to their members. First are understanding and acceptance based on common experience. These lead to better morale. Being able to tell one's troubles to people who understand can be a tonic in itself, especially after perpetually finding incomprehension, ridicule and rejection – which, as we shall see in a later chapter, were not uncommon experiences for respondents. Knowing that one is not the only victim of the affliction and of its institutionalized misrecognition and mishandling can provide a lift for the demoralized. But in addition to invaluable psychosocial care, the groups provide factual information and practical guidelines for applying it. Books, articles, diet sheets, speakers, documentary films become more readily available than they might otherwise be and, if there are questions, someone who has been through a similar experience may be able to advise. The advisory role which members who have sorted themselves out can play is another unique feature of self-help groups and one which received favourable comments from a number of respondents. Through being able to salvage something from their own suffering that is useful to others, group members may be able to find some meaning in what they have been through and their long tribulations may cease to be completely meaningless. We have already heard from Alice A that part of the group's usefulness for her is that, 'I can help others by my experience.' Jennifer H emphasized the value of 'sharing hints', and Joan P, forced into early retirement by her multiple hypersensitivities, said of her group, 'I have been able to help them more than the other way around.'

The attitude of wishing one's suffering to be of benefit to others extended to participation in the survey. In her questionnaire, Veronica S, the mother of an allergic teenager, wrote at the end:

> I do hope this will have been of some help. I would be very pleased if I thought our experience had been of some help to someone else or that life for people with these problems was made somewhat easier through your study.

This concern for the welfare of other sufferers is probably one of the most important features of the groups which, in addition to providing aid and comfort to members, also strive to publicize the condition, the inadequacies in official provisions for meeting sufferers' needs, the environmental conditions that contribute to causing the problem, and the secondary problems which arise for sufferers because of it. Newsletters which circulate to professionals as well as to lay members, talks and conferences, fund-raising events, sponsorship for research and self-generated research are some of the many ways in which the groups promote the cause. But from the individual sufferer's point of view, their most important function is to provide the information, understanding, support and advice that the statutory services seem either unable or unwilling to provide.

In the next three chapters, we will look in more detail at the secondary problems arising from allergy.

7.

Limitations on Everyday Activities Resulting from Allergy

In view of the wide range of allergens the survey group reported and in view of the many self-management activities they adopted to deal with their hypersensitivities, they might reasonably be expected to come up against limitations in their efforts to lead their everyday lives. They were asked to describe any such limitations as follows:

> Do these problems cause you to limit your activities in any way? If so, how (include avoidance of allergenic substances here, as well as avoidance of situations in which exposure to them might occur).

In this chapter we will consider the group's replies to this question.

Distribution of Limitations

The limitations that respondents mentioned were submitted to content analysis without prior attempts at a reductive categorization. This analysis showed that, as in the previous analyses, women mentioned a higher average number of limitations than men: 5.28 (S.D. 4.24) for women, versus 4.50 (S.D. 3.38) for men. They also reported a wider range: 0–28 for women versus 0–12 for men. However, upon inspection it appeared that there was not necessarily a correlation between the number of items mentioned in answer to the question and the overall degree of impairment in the respondent's quality of life. Thus, for example, some respondents wrote flatly that because of their condition they had been unable to live normal lives for some years, but this counted as only one response to the question. Accordingly, a more qualitative system of classifying respondents according to their reported degree of limitation was adopted.

In this system, respondents were placed in one of three categories as follows. Those who reported no limitation and the one lone participant who failed to answer the question were regarded as having no limitations. At the opposite extreme, those who stated or who strongly implied that their ability to pursue normal lives was seriously compromised were regarded as having severe limitation. The remaining respondents were regarded as having some limitation. The results of this analysis are given in Table 31. The table shows that according to this

Table 31:   Degree of limitations mentioned by survey respondents

Category	Males		Females		All	
	n	%	n	%	n	%
Severe limitation	4	20.00	14	21.54	18	21.18
Some limitation	15	75.00	45	69.23	60	70.59
No limitation	1	5.00	5	7.69	6	7.05
No reply	0	0.00	1	1.54	1	1.18

analysis, the proportions of men and women in the three categories are approximately the same. Roughly seventy per cent of the group reported some degree of limitation and twenty-one percent reported severe limitation. The remaining eight percent were not hampered in everyday life by their condition, by their own report. Thus around ninety-two percent of the sample were limited in their daily lives at least to some extent because of their allergies and hypersensitivities.

The next question was whether there was any tendency for those in the three limitation categories to differ in the average number of allergens and symptoms they reported and, for good measure, the absolute number of limitations. These figures are shown in Table 32. The table shows that there is a tendency for people who report limitations to be affected by a wider range of allergens than people who do not report limitations. The number of different types of symptoms, as well as the absolute

Table 32:   Degree of limitation in relation to mean number of
allergens, symptoms and number of limitations

	No limitation (n = 7)	Some limitation (n = 60)	Severe limitation (n = 18)
Allergen categories	3.00	4.63	4.28
Symptom categories	5.86	7.23	10.39
Limitations	0	4.47	8.33

number of limitations also tends to increase with the overall
degree of limitation, but these are only trends. People in the
'severe limitation' category reported a marginally smaller
average number of allergen categories than people in the 'some
limitation' category and there were both 'severely limited'
people with relatively small numbers of symptom types and
particular limitations mentioned and people who qualified as
having only some degree of limitation who reported large
numbers of symptom types and particular limitations.
Although in the group as a whole there can be said to be some
degree of relationship between the degree to which normal life is
precluded and the degree of affectedness in terms of range of
allergens, symptoms, and individual areas of life that are made
difficult by the condition, for any particular individual the
overall degree of social handicap depends on a number of other
factors and cannot necessarily be predicted from bald figures.

The factors that determine the extent to which a person will
be handicapped in everyday activities by an allergic condition
include the nature of the person's self-management regimen for
controlling it as well as on the condition itself, so we need to
consider contributions arising from both sources.

Two important contributors are the nature of the person's
allergens and the frequency with which they are likely to be
encountered in his or her natural environment. These affect the
degree of exposure risk and the extent of the precautionary
measures the person must take to avoid exposure. Thus
someone allergic to, say, poison ivy would be unlikely to be
handicapped by this allergy if living in a place where the plant
didn't grow. By contrast, someone living in Western society
where these foods are basic dietary staples might be seriously
disadvantaged by hypersensitivity to wheat and milk. Someone
who lived in a dusty, old house would have similar problems if
allergic to the house-dust mite.

The nature and severity of the sufferer's symptoms and the degree to which they are intrinsically disabling also obviously make an important contribution. An affliction taking an acute, self-limited and circumscribed form such as a localized rash would probably be less grossly handicapping to most people than continuous prostration, mental confusion or emotional disturbance, and if all three occurred together, so much the worse. But lifestyle and the degree to which it can accommodate a given person's particular types of affliction and regimen are also quite important. A cinema actress or a model for cosmetics might find a facial rash severely limiting, whereas a lighthouse keeper, living in isolation, might find it less of a disaster. Some problems are probably intrinsically more difficult to accommodate than others and some lifestyles more flexible. Intermittent, non-disabling problems will be generally easier to contain and lifestyles with a great deal of leeway for individual timing and choice will probably be better suited to containment. In this context, the stage of life at which problems occur is also critical. The demands which the person's situation places on his or her ability to mix, eat and breathe freely cannot be underestimated. Thus one respondent, an elderly woman retired after an active and demanding professional career and now following a complex rotation diet noted, 'The diet would have been a severe handicap during my professional life and does even now limit my activities and my husband's.' The stage of life may also determine how the handicap operates. A young child whose ability to concentrate was so impaired by hypersensitivity to foods and chemical additives that he couldn't learn to read would be barred from all subsequent learning that presupposes literacy; by contrast a student whose examination performance was handicapped by springtime hay fever might miss out on subsequent opportunities that depended upon doing well in exams but wouldn't be left with a basic skill deficit.

Finally, the affected individual's resources – personal, social, practical and financial – for dealing with the problem also contribute to determining the extent to which it becomes a significant handicap. People who are well endowed with resources will be in a better position to ensure that their affliction remains contained than people who, even without the additional burden, are already struggling against great odds to remain afloat.

Table 33:   Types of limitation mentioned by survey respondents

Category	No. items	Total frequency
Difficult situations	39	137
Avoidance behaviours	14	49
Avoidance strategies	6	38
Physical effects	8	31
Psychological effects	12	30
Social costs	14	24
Economic costs and effects on work	8	18
Effects on family life	4	13
Special problems	4	10
Limits to mobility	4	5
Temporal costs	3	4
Miscellaneous	4	8

In view of the contribution of all these interacting factors and in view of the great diversity of backgrounds and situations of the survey respondents, it is not surprising that there is no uniform, linear relationship between the various indices of affectedness.

Types of Limitation

A broad outline of the overall categories of respondents' limitations, the number of items in each and their respective frequencies are shown in Table 33. From this general outline, it appears that there are a number of different types of experience and activity that respondents regard as either limited or limiting. External situations, people's efforts to avoid their allergens, symptoms of the disorder, and a variety of secondary causes and further symptoms, resulting in one way or another from the condition can all constitute extra burdens for the allergic and hinder their efforts to live ordinary lives. Now let us examine the individual categories in more detail.

Difficult situations

'Difficult situations' are either those in which sufferers experience special problems because of their hypersensitivities or which they must avoid altogether for the same reason. The complete list is given in Table 34. Here we may begin to appreciate the heavy social costs of at least some allergic conditions. It is clear from this list that many of the occasions

Table 34:   Situations causing respondents special difficulty or
which they had to avoid altogether

Situation	f	Situation	f
Eating out	21	Church	2
Social eating/drinking	11	School dinners	1
Parties	9	Formal occasions	1
Meals at others' homes	8	Situations with no control	
Hotels	8	over food choice	1
Holidays	8	Staying in unknown places	1
Restaurants	7	Flying	1
Visiting family, friends	6	Sampling foods	1
Smoky atmospheres	6	Staying late at work	1
Public places (theatre,		Evening class	1
concert, cinema, pub)	6	Swimming	1
Going out socially	5	Washing	1
Business functions	4	Arrangements made in	
Travelling	4	advance	1
Meals, snacks when out for		Noise and commotion	1
day	2	Shopping	1
Summer camp	2	Waiting rooms	1
Buying take-away food	2	Getting hair done	1
Hospitalization	2	Wearing make up	1
Conferences, lectures	2	Playing musical instrument	1
Home entertaining	2	Playing with pets	1
Crowds, crowded places	2		

that provide pleasure and companionable recreation for people who are not allergic may become sources of difficulty and distress for people who are. Those who do not miss out entirely on events such as holidays, eating out, parties, travelling and the like, must go about these activities with extreme circumspection. If they do decide to take the risks inherent in participating, they may face uncertainty about whether the situation will turn out to be safe, knowing that if it doesn't they will most probably become ill. Many supposedly enjoyable events can turn into nightmares. Some reports from respondents will illustrate how ordinary everyday activities can be ruined for victims of the many forms of environmental intolerance.

Joan P, probably the most severely affected of all the survey respondents, suffers from a widespread hypersensitivity to chemical exposure and used to react to foods but has received desensitization to these. In answer to the question on limitations, she gave the following report:

> It has completely taken over my life and that of my husband (he changed his job) in increasing leaps and bounds. I now stay nearly all the time in my bedroom with my air purification machine on night and day and I feel much better. I go out to the sea for a walk with my husband on Sundays, but even there have had attacks. Once a person walked by wearing strong perfume and more recently there appeared to be an invisible barrier at one part of the beach. Later investigations showed why. We hadn't noticed a sign warning of oil and my husband thinks there was detergent as well because the water's edge was covered with thick froth blowing about. . .

Her experience represents an extreme form of the allergic person's typical predicament. Situations and events that are not only safe but even positively beneficial for others are full of hazard and health risk for them. Joan's tale is echoed by Nell F, another sufferer from what we might call total allergy. 'I have become a virtual recluse,' the sixty-four year-old retired woman wrote. 'Having trouble with foods, tobacco smoke, hydrocarbons etc. makes going out a nightmare.' She described a whole range of situations that she is now unable to enter and concluded that this is, 'all very depressing as I used to be the life and soul of the party'.

People do not have to be allergic to virtually everything to have trouble with everyday situations. One or two common allergens are enough to start making life difficult, especially if it isn't always possible or convenient to avoid them. Helen F, a fifty-seven year-old housewife, who suffers from a number of food allergies, wrote, 'staying in hotels can be a nightmare.' Ted J, the asthmatic student with food and hydrocarbon problems that we encountered earlier, is also allergic to cats, which is a bind, since many of his friends have them:

> I cannot sleep in the same room as a cat and prefer not to sleep in a room in which a cat has recently, frequently been. I do in fact sometimes sleep in a room that a cat has spent some time in, but just for one night. This causes my nose to run

and I feel rather stuffy in the head.

Ted's problem illustrates another facet of the difficulty. Allergenic 'contamination' can remain in an environment even after its source has been removed, and an allergic person may not always be able to find out the relevant chapter and verse of history. Even though a visible source of allergen isn't present, the place may still be unsafe. This problem can take a variety of forms, as Sue M's report illustrates. Sue, aged twenty-four, is allergic to eggs in any form:

> I cannot handle eggs or be in the same place when they are being cooked, as this starts off a reaction. I cannot eat food which has been cooked after an egg has been used in the same frying pan unless the pan is washed out thoroughly after cooking the egg.

Tom S, our eczematous young psychologist, made a similar comment about needing to know in which brand of washing powder articles of clothing destined for his use had been washed.

Yet another facet of the difficulty is that the sufferer is faced with invidious choices. Frequently the situation is one in which, whatever he does, he will incur some penalty. Often the dilemma lies between showing socially-expected behaviour and making oneself sick. Some choose to suffer rather than call attention to themselves. Michael S, a retired department store buyer in his sixties, wrote:

> In my younger days I would go to a party and know the price I would have to pay next day – headache. Now I tend to be much stricter and now refuse drinks and sandwiches etc., which is socially a nuisance.

The mother of one hyperactive boy who was badly affected by both gluten and chemical food additives noted that although normally her son had to stick strictly to his diet so that his school work would not be interfered with, 'children's parties obviously require a relaxation of the regimen'. Dierdre E noted that she was unable to avoid a number of difficult social occasions because her husband's job entailed a certain amount of business entertaining. Megan T, a nurse, wrote: 'I dislike the very smoky atmosphere one encounters at social gatherings but see no way to avoid this.'

Not surprisingly, however, many respondents reported opting out of potentially risky activities rather than paying the price in symptoms or subjecting themselves to social pressure to infringe their limitations. Helena Y, a forty-four year-old housewife, reported, 'We can only have self-catering holidays; unable to attend functions involving food and drink.' Bernice W, a forty-nine year-old office worker mentioned that she hadn't attended a Christmas dinner party, not only because she couldn't afford the ticket but also because, 'I couldn't have eaten it all anyway.' She reported that she has stayed away from other office gatherings because of these problems. Brian G, whom we heard from earlier, said that 'all food is prepared by either my wife or myself'; he regarded this as 'a severe handicap to social life'. But, as Sarah V, a thirty-five year-old lecturer, noted at the end of a long list of social and business functions that she couldn't attend since they involved the possibility of exposure to allergenic foods: 'This is very limiting, but I can't afford the time or stress involved in having major reactions.' For some, the price of participation is too steep.

Avoidance Tactics and Strategies
In view of the widespread risk of exposure to common allergens and environmental pollutants in everyday life, it is not surprising that avoidance strategies and tactics were frequently mentioned. The results of this analysis are shown in Table 35.

Manoeuvres to avoid both foods and chemicals loom large in this list; avoidance of organic non-food allergens was not so often mentioned as a general formulation. It is clear from the list of particular avoidance behaviours that many different forms of activity are likely to be involved in implementing the general strategies and that in some cases considerable inconvenience and possible social embarrassment may be entailed. Thus Sue M wrote:

> I'm not all that keen on dining out, either in restaurants or at people's houses unless I know them very well. It can be very embarrassing always having to ask if such and such has any egg in it, especially if it's a pretty formal kind of occasion.

In a similar vein, Janet I a twenty-five year-old writer, said that

Table 35:   Avoidance behaviours and strategies

Behaviours–category	f	Strategies–category	f
Bring own food along	11	Avoid allergenic foods	22
Take care in choosing food	6	Avoid noxious indoor environments	7
Self-catering holidays	5	Avoid chemical inhalants	4
Meals only with close friends	4	Avoid situations of possible exposure to allergens	2
Refuse food offered	3	Avoid contact with allergenic substances (skin)	2
Prepare own food	3		
Get information re ingredients	3		
Forewarn hosts, hostesses, etc.	3	Avoid animals	1
Decline invitations	3		
Leave early to avoid smoke	2		
Find safe cooking utensils	2		
Home baking	1		
Find safe seats	1		
Find unscented cosmetics	1		
Find safe food (in shops)	1		

although people co-operate with keeping their cats and dogs out of her way, they 'appear sometimes to resent this'. Whatever sufferers do, they are likely to have trouble. Mike P, the young doctor with allergy to peppers, noted that he sometimes experienced difficulty in extracting information about ingredients from waiters and that sometimes he had to resort to threatening to sue the establishment if they got the information wrong before it was forthcoming.

The typical pattern of respondents' experiences in trying to live with their condition involves both the loss of desirable opportunities and the acquisition of many undesirable additional burdens. This pattern will become clearer in the next sections, which document more of the hidden costs of being allergic.

Physical Costs
Physical effects of their condition were reported by numerous respondents under the general heading of limitations. They are shown in Table 36. Even if the sufferer is not incapacitated by acute symptoms resulting from unavoidable exposures, he or she may live in a state of perpetual low-grade debilitation due to chronic malnutrition, adrenal exhaustion and generally decreased resistance to stress. Brian G's report epitomizes this problem:

The most persistent symptoms have been mental and physical fatigue, so that very little is done apart from doing what I can at work. We have moved into a flat, purchased a car with automatic transmission, employed tradesmen in place of do-it-yourself and done all possible to streamline essential activity. Some of the difficulties may arise from long periods of inadequate diet.

As a result of this state of reduced vitality, some sufferers are likely to have to miss out on social and recreational activities that would be safe from the point of view of allergies, simply because they haven't got enough energy left to participate. Thus Marge E, a fifty-one year-old housewife with widespread food allergies, wrote, 'I haven't felt fit enough for the past ten years to lead a normal life.' Elizabeth T, a fifty-one year-old housewife, also afflicted with multiple food allergies, wrote that her difficulties didn't limit her activities generally, 'but if I have had a bad reaction then I would have to stay at home for a while'. She continued:

I have led quite an active life (in spite of these problems and even before I discovered it was allergy) but it has been hard work to keep going and I do wonder what life would have been like if I had not been thus afflicted. I think I would have had a lot more energy.

Some are not as fortunate as Elizabeth in being able to carry on. Esther W, a sixty-three year-old housewife, wrote, 'I live a very quiet life. Avoid all entertaining and excursions out. All too fatiguing. I get so terribly tired very easily.' And Polly U, a

Table 36:   Physical costs of allergic conditions

Category	f
Symptoms from being unable to avoid allergens	8
Limited diet	7
Weakness, fatigue, reduced energy	7
Interference with exercise, sports	5
Increased physical vulnerability	1
Symptoms disfiguring	1
Need for excessive sleep	1
Problems secondary to inadequate diet	1

forty-three year-old housewife, described a vicious circle:

> I get overtired easily and this lowers my allergy tolerance level. . . I try to live a quiet life. With three lively children, a fit husband and a very exuberant dog, however, this is virtually impossible.

Karen D, a nurse in her early thirties afflicted with chemical and food problems, wrote simply, 'I feel like sleeping all the time.' And Helena Y, a forty-four year-old housewife, reported that 'lack of energy and depression inhibit normal daily life'. The general debilitation resulting from chronic allergy is not generally appreciated except by those who have to live with it.

Psychological Costs
As Helena's and Brian's reports suggest, the physical deficits resulting from allergic conditions have their psychological counterparts too. Nearly as many of the limitations that were mentioned came under this heading. They are shown in Table 37.

Table 37:   Psychological costs of allergic conditions

Category	f
Self consciousness, embarrassment	7
Depression	5
Mental confusion	4
Loss of pleasure	3
Frustration	2
Restricted activity	2
Interference of symptoms with mental functioning	2
Food choice dictated by rota	1
Temptation	1
Dread of eating	1
Interference with independence	1
Lowering of self-esteem	1

In some cases, as in Helena's and Brian's reports, physical and psychological costs were linked. This was also the case in Tom S's report, though the relationship was different. Tom's eczematous shins led him to give the following account:

> I am occasionally embarrassed, e.g. on a beach or at a

sporting event where my shins are exposed, particularly if they are looking raw. People staring at your deformity is not very pleasant.

But it is not only physical symptoms which have the effect of making allergic people conspicuous. Mental confusion and woolliness can have the same impact. Alan B, the young chemical victim whose tale we heard earlier, wrote, 'People may think you are odd if they notice you are sometimes anxious and confused and other times not so.' Helen F, a migraine sufferer, noted: 'Never being sure of being able to keep a date and having to decline taking on responsibilities for fear of letting people down is devastating to oneself and difficult to explain to others.'

People can also feel singled out by their regimens of avoidance. Thus Marie L, a sixty year-old retired social worker, described her situation:

> I rather dread social occasions when I may be invited to eat things that cause me problems. I feel self-conscious about these things, especially if people around me can eat what they like.

This problem was particularly acute for children, who seem generally to have an aversion to being different but who often had to be sent to parties with a packed supply of their own safe food.

Self-consciousness, embarrassment and loss of self-esteem are only part of the psychological cost of allergies. In addition, many respondents reported that their afflictions interfered directly with their mental functioning and thus limited what they could do. Thus Bernice W wrote, 'With my head so muddled I don't think I could learn new skills or relearn old unused skills.' The contest of her statement was a quandary about her work. Alan B said, 'I find it impossible to work properly when anxious and confused.' Henry J, a twenty-six year old student, mentioned depression 'and constant churning over of thoughts non-stop (rumination) and the inability to concentrate that results' as constituting serious problems for him. And Sarah V, a lecturer with multiple food and chemical problems resulting in migraines and a state of mental fuzziness, remarked, 'It's hard to think or do anything when your head feels full of cotton wool.'

Table 38:   Social costs of allergic conditions

Category	f
Interference with sociability and relationships	5
Precludes normal life	4
Pressure to join in	3
Uncertainty about keeping appointments	2
Disposing of unwanted food	1
Having to explain to others	1
Having to ask for special food	1
Interference with taking on responsibilities	1
Interference with helping others	1
Increased isolation	1
Not invited out	1
Interference with education	1
Letting others down	1
Being misunderstood	1

These poignant reports highlight some of the hidden costs to sufferers of their strange afflictions. They are only the tip of the iceberg, as we shall see in the next section concerning the social costs of allergies.

Social Costs

The social costs of allergy shown in Table 38, were also heavy. The most frequent complaint was that the sufferer's condition interfered with social relationships. One young woman reported that she had lost several boyfriends because they got fed up with her being ill all the time. A young man complained that his food-induced mental symptoms led to 'total inability to have healthy emotional relationships with anyone'. He described a phobia of social situations as one of his symptoms. Another woman wrote, 'The depression causes avoidance of social contact with other people.' They are not the only ones. Four people reported that their condition virtually precluded normal life – including most everyday social relationships. A single-parent head of family, raising four children on her own against great odds, wrote, 'This problem isolates me even more than I am already.'

But others, who were able to participate to a greater extent, had the added burden of social pressure to join in and be like everybody else – despite the fact, as we saw earlier, that this would involve the risk of exposure to some of their allergens.

Judith I, a forty-eight year-old housewife, spoke for others when she wrote, 'I cannot drink alcohol, which makes me stand out rather: "But you must have a drink!"' Some people, like Eleanor B, a forty year-old housewife, take their own food to parties or else just eat a little of anything that doesn't upset them. Those who give into the pressure either, like Michael S in his younger days, pay the price in symptoms the next day, or, like Sylvia K, a thirty-six year-old psychologist, accept the forbidden food and then 'hide it or persuade my husband to drink/eat it instead'.

From these reports it appears that social events take on a new dimension of meaning for many allergic people. Occasions that others tend to view as opportunities for enjoyable participation can come to seem like obstacle courses, fraught with hazards both obvious and hidden. The magnitude of threat varies with the nature of the sufferer's sensitivities and the particulars of the occasion, but some degree of threat is usually present. At one extreme, social situations can lead to incapacitating symptoms. Joan P, for example, the total-allergy victim we met earlier, described how she was once visited at home by a member of the allergy club to which she belongs. Her acquaintance turned up wearing 'masses of perfume'. Joan said that she was crying within a short time and had to be put to bed and given oxygen. At the other extreme is Jenny M's report of the effects of hypersensitivity to caffeine on her social life: 'It doesn't really stop me doing anything socially, but does slightly spoil things like going out to dinner, etc. when everyone else is having coffee at the end.' In between these two extremes, environmental hypersensitivity may mean that a party is something you leave halfway through because of the smoke, a hostess is someone you forewarn that you'll be bringing your own food, and a conference is somewhere you can't attend because of the air conditioning. Moreover, as we shall in the following chapter, it means that you are someone very few others may understand.

Economic Costs and Effects on Work
In addition to the more intangible physical, psychological and social costs, allergy may bring with it a number of concrete economic costs, which correspond to the now familiar pattern of loss of advantages and gain of disadvantages. The items included under this heading are given in Table 39.

Table 39:   Economic costs and effects on work

Category	f
Safe food costs more	4
Problems interfere with work	4
Precludes work outside home	2
Limits activities to essentials	2
Change of residence	2
Replacement of equipment	2
Hired help	1
Problems secondary to being unable to work	1

The loss side of the account centres on interference with the ability to hold a job, which leads to reduced earning capacity, as suggested in the following reports. Hazel S, a thirty-four year-old assistant accountant who suffers from hypoglycaemia, described her situation: 'As I have to eat at 3–3½ hour intervals I am unable to do the work I would like, as not many employers would understand or tolerate my disappearing every few hours to eat.'

Rita M, a forty-six year-old self-employed woman, suffers from allergies to a range of common foods. Her story is similar:

I would find it difficult to go out to work full time. It does help working from home. I always have to carry a snack and plant milk with me.

Dierdre E, a fifty-four year-old housewife, also reported that, 'I couldn't hold down a part-time job' because of her widespread food and chemical sensitivities. Sheila O, forty-eight, a teacher with similar afflictions, wrote that her allergies, 'made me so ill that eventually I did no work and had vast problems'. Andrea A, the multi-allergic house-wife whose story we heard earlier on, wrote: 'When I make a mistake and eat some form of my allergens unsuspectingly, it makes me very ill so I can't do anything other than the absolute essentials.' And Eileen J, from whom we also heard earlier, noted that her diet would have been 'a severe handicap during my professional life'.

From these accounts it is plain that sufferers can have their working capacity interfered with, not only by their symptoms but also by the regimens they are obliged to adopt in order to control them. Not only the quantity but also the quality of work can be impaired, as Jessica T, twenty-six, noted. Before sorting out her diet, she observed, 'my work was not as good as it is now'. For others, limited aspects of work were compromised. Sarah V reported that 'staying late at work and business lunches are out'. She regarded this as 'very limiting'. Several others also mentioned these limitations.

On the side of gains of undesirable burdens, respondents emphasized the additional expenses incurred through their allergies. The increased cost of 'safe' food – which in one case was reported to be prohibitive – was the most frequent comment. As mentioned earlier, one mother of a hyperactive boy noted that he is 'very expensive to feed – £2.50 per day on average' – and that was in 1979. In addition to increased food costs, some people had the extra expense of replacing allergenic household equipment and in a few cases of a complete move of house. Extra equipment for purifying the atmosphere could also be expensive, as Joan P's report suggests:

Bought water purification unit, stainless steel saucepans, kitchen extractor, American air purification unit and personal one, oxygen. Moved near the sea and removed gas, nylon, and plastic as much as I am able. . . Got a shower unit as a bath takes too long and sends me off with the chlorine. . . Got a cast-iron bath instead of plastic. Only electric heating, etc.

Brian G's similar activities have already been described. They were undertaken in order to streamline his life and reduce his need to expend energy, but the resulting extra expense is the same – a complete move of house, purchase of a new car, use of tradesmen in place of do-it-yourself, and so on. Another woman said she was about to exchange her gas cooker for an electric one but hadn't done so yet. None mentioned any outside financial help with their extra expenses, but one woman did say that she had heard of a trust that sometimes might contribute towards helping people with such additional expenditures incurred through their illness.

Although respondents did not mention the cost of private treatment under the heading of limitations, several did comment upon this additional expense in giving their answers to other questions. In one case the context was that the treatment had been more than the respondent could afford.

From these reports it appears that one of the many hidden

Table 40:   Effects of allergic conditions on home and family life

Category	f
Interference with activities of other family members	6
Interference with household chores	3
Supervision of child staying away from home	2
Limits to family size	2

handicaps of allergy is the invidious combination of reduced ability to earn a living and the extra expenses involved in ensuring day-to-day survival.

Effects on Home and Family Life

In view of the wide range of problems that sufferers have so far reported, we should expect there to be reports of detrimental effects of allergic conditions on home and family life. There were and these are shown in Table 40.

Although relatively few items were mentioned, those that were represented a profound degree of interference in normal social life, as may be seen in the following report from the mother of Jason, a hyperactive toddler:

> Hyperactive behaviour of the child rules the whole family. Jason will not sit still for shopping, eating, or [in] waiting rooms for long. His energy wears me out and the frustration in him means he is difficult to handle. I do not take him on outings too much because I am embarrassed by his behaviour. Because he is only twenty months I can control his diet. I take his own drink when out and most people have a plain biscuit in the house if they must insist on giving him something. I have to read all the labels on food products. Even in a health-food shop there are some preservatives in the foods.

She added a painful description of her feelings for her son:

> Although I love my son, I do not enjoy looking after him. Most people can control their children's behaviour. We can't. We are afraid of having more children. All we can do is muddle through the day and hope that with the support of the Feingold Diet Jason will improve as he gets older. I worry that I will not be able to cope with him.

This mother's fear of having more children is not an isolated instance. Two other women said that their allergic condition made them decide either to remain childless, despite the desire to have children eventually, or to refrain from having any more. 'I know I couldn't cope with a baby with my problems,' wrote one of the women. And another declared, 'Thank goodness I won't be having any more children to pass it [the condition] on to.' Although allergy *per se* probably does not reduce fertility at a biological level, it may lead to a reproductive disadvantage for the afflicted. This is a point that does not seem to be widely appreciated.

The presence of an affected member may impair the quality of family life for all. Spouses may be restricted by their partner's dietary restrictions, chemical sensitivities, and inability to mix. They may have to take on extra chores because their partner is too exhausted to do more than a bare minimum or must avoid contact with allergens or is off in the loo being sick. If an affected child stays overnight away from home, the mother may have to stay with him to supervise his diet. Children may have to miss out on favourite activities because their parents cannot participate. Thus Reg R wrote that because of his hypersensitivity to water he never goes swimming any more, 'much to the annoyance of my young boys'. Thus at all levels, from procreation to recreation, the restrictive effects of environmental hypersensitivity in one member of the family can spread to others.

Limits to Mobility

Even the basic capacity to move freely in space may be compromised by allergy or by the means adopted to control it. The items mentioned by respondents under this heading, which are shown in Table 41, show the usual pattern of lost advantages and acquired disadvantages. Two respondents complained that whenever they went anywhere for the day or longer, they were laden with containers and utensils for

Table 41:   Limits to mobility resulting from allergic conditions

Category	f
Burden of food containers and equipment	2
Interference with going out of doors	2
Having to come home for lunch	1

reparing their special diet foods. Others were prevented from
going out of doors because of susceptibility to airborne
inhalants and other menaces: 'It [pollen and insect sensitivity]
puts one off the great outdoors generally,' wrote one woman.
One young man reported that he chose *not* to avoid going out of
doors in the pollen season because he would mind the absence
of sunshine more than he minded his hay-fever symptoms.
Finally, the mother of one school-age hyperactive child reported
that her youngster had to come home for lunch because the
school had a regulation that children who didn't take the school
dinners could not bring their own packed lunches and stay at
school. Sometimes the rules seem to be made especially to
create additional disadvantages for already-handicapped
allergic people.

Temporal Costs

Surprisingly few respondents mentioned the extra time their
condition demanded and the responses pertaining to this aspect
of the problems of being allergic are shown in Table 42. The

Table 42:   Temporal costs of allergic conditions

Category	f
Time spent planning	2
Shopping takes longer	1
Reactions are time-consuming	1

respondents who mentioned time spent planning all referred to
the same basic problem: how to organize their regimens. Thus
if people go out for the day they may need to work out how
much safe food they are going to need for the time they will be
away; how they are going to carry it, prevent if from going off
without refrigeration; where they are going to be able to
consume it, and so forth. Shopping for safe food or other goods
may take longer than ordinary shopping, since it may require
trips to a number of different shops that are not all in the same
locality. And if sufferers incur a severe reaction they may be
incapacitated for days at a time. Other respondents, whose
reports were coded under different headings, reported losing
time through their need for extra sleep and through being able
to do only the barest essentials.
   Although relatively few respondents alluded to the temporal

costs of their condition, the impact of this lost time on an affected person can be considerable. It is possible that these aspects of the problem of living with allergy were not mentioned in proportion to their functional importance because sufferers tend to habituate to the waste of time their state entails and come to take the extra demands it places upon them for granted.

Special Problems

In addition to the various costs of allergy, survey participants also mentioned a number of special problems which they regarded as limitations arising from it; these are given in Table 43. Difficulties which people reported in keeping to their

Table 43:   Special problems of allergic people

Category	f
Difficulty sticking to regimen	5
Unavoidability of allergen exposure	2
Difficulty detecting culprits	2
Over-reliance on Nalcrom	1

regimens of allergen avoidance mainly resulted from situational factors, but in one case the cause was the sufferer's habit of binge eating. The two cases who reported that exposure to their allergens was impossible to avoid were both hypersensitive to the cigarette smoke encountered at social gatherings. Two others said that they were hampered by inability conclusively to indentify their food precipitants, which meant that they could not effectively avoid them and hence were liable to develop symptoms. Finally, one woman complained of leaning too heavily on Nalcrom. These reports appeared to refer to limitations on regimen-following behaviour and suggest, collectively, that for sufferers regimen-following tends to become an ordinary everyday activity.

To summarize the findings about limitations, we may say that there seems to be practically no area of ordinary social life that allergy or hypersensitivity to foods or other environmental factors doesn't interfere with for someone. Work, sociability, leisure, exercise, sport, education, family life, church, cultural participation, pets, musical performance, hygiene, grooming, mobility, nutrition, even reproduction – all can be ruined for somebody. Not all allergic sufferers are impaired equally across all areas, but only a few – under ten percent – escape without some impairment of their capacity to lead normal lives. The pattern of affectedness typically involves both missing out on normal opportunities and having to contend with a variety of extra problems and worries. Many difficulties may interact with each other: reduced earning capacity with increased expenses, reduced energy with extra preparation needed to secure safe operating conditions, increased isolation with reduced self-esteem. Whichever way we look at it, we find that allergic people tend to suffer numerous social, psychological and practical handicaps in addition to whatever basic biological predisposition causes them to react adversely to their allergens. One disadvantage breeds another in a vicious downward spiral.

In the following chapter we will examine some of the social handicaps incurred by allergic people in more detail.

8.

Social Reactions to Allergic People

Robinson and Henry noted that one of the important characteristics of 'abnormal' problems was that people who do not have them tend to look down on people who do. In this chapter we will examine survey respondents' reports of their experience of other people's reactions to them and their difficulties. This discussion may be seen as a contribution to the small but growing literature on public stereotypes of the chronically ill[1], but the method adopted to explore the question of how allergic people appear in the public eye differs from the one which is usually employed.

Normally, an investigator asks a group of non-affected people about their views of a particular group of afflicted people. While this approach may yield information about public stereotypes, it doesn't tell us much about a perhaps more important question, namely, what it is like for sufferers to be on the receiving end of these schematic and often extremely distorted views. To answer this question, we need to obtain information directly from the afflicted group; to ask them how they perceive others as perceiving them. If common trends appear in the independent reports of many, we may discount the possibility of individual bias in sufferers' perceptions of how other people regard them.

This latter procedure was followed in the present study. Two analyses were carried out, one concerning respondents' direct reports of how others tend to react to them and a second concerning derogatory labels or terms of abuse which they mentioned in any context as either having been applied to them or people like them or which they feared would be applied if they were to call attention to their special difficulties. Let us now examine each of these topics in turn.

Social Reactions

For this analysis, respondents were asked about other people's reactions to them as follows:

Do you find that people you come into contact with (such as family, friends, relatives, hosts/hostesses/guests, waiters, stewardesses, doctors, nurses, other professionals, etc.) tend to understand these sorts of problems or do you run into misunderstandings? Have there been any particularly outstanding incidents or misunderstandings that stick in your mind?

Their responses were analysed according to the basic categories 'professional' vs. 'lay' and 'understand' vs. 'don't understand' or in more general terms such as 'incident mentioned'. The results of this analysis are shown in Table 44, where it will be seen that the percentages add up to more than 100 percent because responses were not mutually exclusive and many respondents gave more than one.

Table 44:   Social responses to respondents' problems

Category	f	%
Lay people don't understand	50	58.82
Lay people do understand	36	42.35
Professionals don't understand	32	37.65
Incident mentioned	16	18.82
Professionals do understand	13	15.29
Difficulties mentioned	12	14.12
Misunderstandings–general	5	5.88
No misunderstandings	5	5.88
No reply	2	2.35

From these findings it appears that the majority of respondents encountered at least some degree of social misunderstanding and that on the whole they were more likely to report coming up against incomprehension than sympathy, tolerance and concern, especially when in contact with medical and paramedical professionals.

If the four response categories 'lay do/don't' and 'professionals do/don't' are taken separately, we have eighty-six responses referring to lay people, of which 58.14 percent describe misunderstanding. This suggests that, on the whole, lay people may be somewhat more likely to misunderstand than to understand the problems of allergic people. By contrast, we have forty-five responses referring to professionals and seventy-one percent of these refer to misunderstandings. This suggests that sufferers, by their own reckoning, have about one chance in four of meeting with comprehension in their contacts with members of the various service professions, especially health professionals. In this context it is probably significant that thirteen of the sixteen incidents mentioned took place in medical settings.

The finding that our respondents reported meeting with more understanding from members of the lay public than from doctors, nurses and other professionals seems to reflect two trends. The first is for health professionals to be rigidly prejudiced in their views about patients with multiple complaints who do not have the excuse of having just been run over by a bus. In the course of their professional socialization – which Durkheim has aptly characterized as their 'déformation professionelle' – health workers acquire by precept a number of rules of thumb for dealing with multisymptomatic people, especially those who do not get better on routine management. Needless to say, these rules of thumb are bereft of any acknowledgement of the possibility that such patients are not making up their problems for purposes of being deliberately awkward[2]. Lacking the benefits of an expensive medical education, members of the lay public have not been institutionally programmed to reject the allergic out of hand simply as a matter of principle.

Secondly, the greater understanding shown by lay people reflects the recent effort by the media to raise British consciousness of the existence and nature of food and chemical hypersensitivities, which, as we have noted earlier, was sparked off by the appearance of Mackarness's *Not All in the Mind* in 1976. Several respondents referred appreciatively to the influence of the media in increasing others' tolerance and understanding of their difficulties. Thus Rachel N, a twenty-three year-old secretary, wrote:

I have found that people lack understanding and have been very intolerant. Doctors said it was 'Mind over Body'. During the last two years it has improved a little owing to publicity in women's magazines, radio, television and Dr Mackarness's book. Some relatives have been difficult and ridiculed me.

Nancy D, twenty-seven, gave a similar report:

When I first found out that I suffered from food allergies very few people knew anything about it and there were *many* misunderstandings. Just lately, however, people are much more receptive to the idea due to a great deal of publicity. I also find it easier to tell people about my problems as I have gained confidence in myself.

And Helen F, fifty-seven, wrote: 'People have become more aware of migraine in recent years, thanks to the media, and do tend to be more sympathetic.' But Margaret L, thirty-four, lamented the fact that some people remain unreceptive to the publicity:

Some well-meaning relatives say 'allergy is all in the mind'. They should read the book by Richard Mackarness. If one sees a reaction, it should be regarded with more sympathy by outsiders. One has to live with it to really understand.

Margaret's use of the phrase 'allergy is all in the mind' and her reference to Mackarness's contrapuntal title points up the nature of the revolution in sensibility that seems to be in progress. We now need to consider this development in more detail because it is an important factor in the social reception of allergic people and their difficulties.

The view that 'allergy is all in the mind' represents a popular paradigm, in Kuhn's sense,[3] for the social construction of allergic reactions and those who have them. The origins of this notion are obscure but they most probably include watered-down versions of dicta formulated by the leaders of the psychosomatic movement in earlier twentieth century medicine. Probably as the result of the propagation of the notion that psychological stimuli can trigger symptoms in some people, it has come to be widely assumed, both by many members of the lay public and even more entrenchedly by many members of the medical profession that all symptoms arise by this means unless proven otherwise. Within this procrustean paradigm, the environment is the very last place on earth where symptoms are considered to originate. The main cause is thought to be a deviation of the sufferer's personality, which may take a number of different possible forms: an assumed masochistic desire to suffer; a wish to attract attention; or 'anxiety', a global construct adopted for purposes of writing off instances that cannot conveniently be accommodated by the other categories. Often the symptoms attributed to 'anxiety' are not those normally associated with over-arousal of the sympathetic nervous system: sudden tiredness after a meal, extreme abdominal bloating, constipation, blocked nose without a cold or hay fever, swollen and painful joints – to name but a few – are all within this paradigm routinely attributed to the individual's 'nerves'.

The chief rationale of this paradigm is invalidation of the sufferer's claim to legitimate distress and the extensions of the paradigm, to be discussed below, receive their intelligibility from this underlying *raison d'être*. Before examining the extensions of the 'allergy is all in the mind' paradigm, let us take a look at some reports from respondents that support the argument so far. Other respondents besides Margaret alluded to the stereotype in their answers to the social reaction question. Twenty-six year-old Henry J, for example, wrote that, 'on the whole people are tolerant' but noted that, 'some do think it is "all in the mind"'. Rachel N, twenty-three, said, 'I have found that people lack understanding and have been very intolerant. Doctors said it was "Mind over Body".' Sue M, twenty-four, wrote, 'Most seem to think it's all in the mind and that it is a way of craving for attention.' As Sue's report indicates, respondents also hinted broadly at the main forms of assumed personality deviation that are held responsible for their symptoms. Reg R, forty-three, noted that, 'The apparent opinion is that I *enjoy* bad health and won't eat proper food.' Besides attention-seeking and masochism, 'anxiety' also appeared in respondents' reports. Doreen W, fifty-eight, described the following incident in hospital:

Some years ago I had a gall bladder X-ray. When the nurse gave me the milky-looking drink to take, I warned her I passed out on milky drinks. She assured me it wasn't. Within a few minutes I was flat on the floor. They then said I was scared of having the X-ray.

It may well be that the drink contained no milk. But it most probably did contain egg, to which Doreen is also allergic, and as she reported earlier in the questionnaire could cause her to pass out within minutes of eating.[4] The absurdity of blaming her faint on 'being scared of having the X-ray' is revealed by the fact that in the procedure described, the X-ray taken after the milky drink is the last in a series, none of which seems to have frightened the lady out of her wits. From these reports it is clear that my construction corresponds to the experience reported by survey respondents when encountering the view that 'allergy is all in the mind'.

The main extensions of this basic premise include the following:

1   Sufferers are imagining their symptoms.
2   They exaggerate their imaginary discomfort.
3   Therefore they are obviously mentally unstable ('neurotic', 'hysterical', 'hypochondriacal', etc.) and must under no circumstances be taken seriously.

Let us now examine these propositions in more detail.

Within the peculiar rationality of the 'allergy is all in the mind' paradigm, the causal link between environmental irritants and the development of symptoms is automatically denied. But often the paradigm goes further than this: not only the cause but also the effect is declared to exist only in the sufferer's imagination. Thus Helen Y, forty-four, wrote, 'Relatives can't comprehend the problem and tend to feel it is imagination.' Nell F, sixty-four, wrote that her daughter and others 'think it's "psychological", i.e. "pull yourself together"'. And Pat Z, fifty-eight, said that her doctor once sagely delivered himself of the opinion, 'If you don't think about it, it will go away.' Interestingly, and perhaps not fortuitously, all three of these respondents were middle-aged women whose 'age', as we saw in an earlier chapter, may, like their 'nerves', be used to explain away anything they may feel is wrong with them. By means of such attributions, the legitimacy of sufferers' claims to occupying the sick role[5] is undermined and any dispensation from normal social roles and their attendant responsibilities they receive in recognition of their indisposition is on sufferance rather than as part of a normative system of reciprocal obligations. The lack of appropriate facilities for dealing with sufferers' problems also contributes to the view that they are unreal: after all, if they weren't imaginary, there would be clinics to deal with them, wouldn't there? This extension applies in particular to symptoms that are subjective, such as pain, malaise, fatigue and so forth, where the only evidence for their existence an outsider may have is the sufferer's report.

In cases where objective evidence for the existence of the symptom is unequivocal, the reality basis for the sufferer's complaints cannot so readily be denied. In such cases, the victim's pretensions to legitimate suffering are invalidated by reference to the notion of 'exaggeration' or 'making a fuss over nothing'. Thus nineteen year-old Paul R, a student with multiple, mainly respiratory, allergies, wrote:

> On the whole, people tend to dismiss suffering as minor. Some GPs are particularly unhelpful, refusing to give aid until very ill indeed.

Sue M, twenty-four, so violently allergic to even a minute trace of egg that she cannot use egg shampoo, has constant difficulty avoiding egg as an ingredient in composite dishes and on numerous occasions has required emergency treatment in casualty: 'Most people tend to think you are exaggerating, especially doctors,' she reported. Pat Z, whose sleep is chronically impaired by difficulty in breathing, also wrote: 'Most people I meet greatly underestimate the problem, brushing it aside as "only catarrh". And Marie L, sixty, remarked: 'I have always had the feeling that doctors and people in general seem to think that people are neurotic if they fuss over these things.' In the context of my argument, it is necessary to agree that Marie's perception seems entirely accurate; it is the stereotype that is distorted. The end-result of invalidation by appeals to 'exaggeration' or 'making a fuss' is the same as in the case of refusal to acknowledge the reality of subjective complaints: the sufferer is regarded as inauthentic and gets no sympathy for his/her pains because of being thought to make immoderate claims for them.

The form which this invalidation takes, as Robinson and

Henry noted in their discussion of 'abnormal' problems,[6] is an attitude of stigmatization, in particular, as Marie pointed out, an invocation of the notion of mental disorder. Within the rationality of the 'all in the mind' paradigm, people who have allergies are regarded as not having had the sense not to – they are seen as having in some measure lost their senses. They are *non compos mentis* and accordingly needn't be taken with full seriousness. This socially sanctioned method of 'explaining' sufferers' problems effectively disposes of their credibility. The fact that the method is based on pure assumptions and involves a tautology of the first order of magnitude (allergy is all in the mind, therefore allergic people are mental) is overlooked and the imputed mental pathology stipulated as the cause of allergic symptoms and suffering assumes the status of a fact given in nature. Here the consequences for the sufferer are not only the loss of legitimate consideration in respect of his/her allergic difficulties but also the unwelcome acquisition of a stereotyped deviant social identity.

As we shall consider in greater detail later in this chapter, many respondents alluded to psychopathological labels used as terms of abuse in many contexts throughout the questionnaire. A selection from their reports shows a dismaying degree of stereotypy:

People do not understand and assume I am finicky, neurotic and anorexic. (Alan B, aged thirty three).

Friends try to understand, not always successfully. Doctors tend not to. They assume I'm hypochondriacal. (Sarah V, aged thirty five).

Not much [understanding]. I am seen as faddy, fussy, overprotective, a nuisance generally. (Beverley C, aged forty-seven).

People are generally very interested, but professionals think you're a neurotic food faddist/fanatic. (John M, aged twenty-six).

No one understands. Everyone labels you as neurotic, including doctors. I called a doctor out one night and he told my parents I was a 'psychopath'. (Karen D, aged thirty-three).

People seem to think we are mad eating what we eat. (Rosina K, aged thirty-two).

Misunderstandings!! Suggestion that I'm manic-depressive has stuck. (Dominique D, aged twenty-six).

Whatever the particular terminology used to brand the sufferer a victim of functional psychopathology, the net result of the application of the 'allergy is all in the mind' paradigm is that both he/she and his/her suffering are dismissed as being of no consequence, something they should either 'stop thinking about' or 'learn to live with – a phrase which was widely used throughout the questionnaire.

However, it appears from some respondents' reports that this destructive and damaging paradigm is now being challenged by an alternative approach to construing the nature of allergic people's difficulties. This view, as epitomized in the lapidary title of Mackarness's book, is that 'allergy is *not* all in the mind', but rather arises in an orderly fashion from a concatenation of knowable physical circumstances. The work of the clinical ecologists heralds a revolution in both popular and medical sensibility which may be seen to bear a certain family resemblance to the revolution in the understanding of epilepsy brought about by the Hippocratic manifesto, 'The Sacred Disease'.[7] In this classical text, Hippocrates argued that the popular superstitions about epilepsy were mistaken: 'I do not believe that the ''Sacred Disease'' is any more divine or sacred than any other disease but, on the contrary, has specific characteristics and a definite cause.' The difference between the Hippocratic revolution and the present one is that in the case of allergy the 'new' paradigm really represents a reinstatement of the pre-psychosomatic understanding of the condition. For milennia the fact that certain people reacted adversely to foods and other substances which did not appear to have bad effects on most people was accepted as an empirical fact and those to whom these unusual reactions occurred were not supposed to be merely pretending to experience them. In the more 'enlightened' era of psychosomatic presumption,[8] however, it has become necessary to re-establish the basic principle that sufferers are not inventing their complaints, not exaggerating their distress, and not *de facto* mentally ill, either. Thus T. G. Randolph, a pioneer of clinical ecology, saw fit to dedicate his recent popular introduction to the subject:

. . . to all patients who have ever been called neurotic,

hypochondriacal, hysterical, or starved for attention, while actually suffering from environmentally induced illness.[9]

Like the title of Mackarness's book, Randolph's dedication epitomizes the paradigm shift which appears to be occurring.

However, at the present time the new paradigm for the construction of allergy is still unfortunately far from being universally accepted. The form which rejection of it assumes may be termed scepticism. 'Scepticism' in this context is a mental attitude of rejection. What is rejected is the sufferer's contention that environmental factors are making him ill and that avoidance of these factors produces improvement. A large number of respondents reported encountering this stance:

My good friends are sympathetic and others sceptical. Also most doctors are sceptical. (Andrea A, aged sixty-three).

One old-fashioned doctor was very intolerant and sceptical. (Michael S, aged sixty-nine).

Medical profession are sceptical to say the least. (Paula S, aged sixteen).

Bar family and relatives, most people tend to be sceptical. . . Doctors and nurses are especially sceptical. (Megan T, aged forty-one).

People. . . are a bit sceptical about allergies. (Rosina K, aged thirty-two).

The only scepticism has come from a Harley Street consultant physician and another consultant. (Jennifer H, aged sixty-one)

People who suffer similar queer things are always ready to swop tales but non-sufferers tend to be sceptical. (Mother of Anna W, aged fifteen)

Non-medical friends and family have been sympathetic. Medicals – one doctor friend has no time for it at all. Of my two GPs, one is open-minded and quite interested, the other thinks it irrelevant. (Sally C, aged twenty-four)

Encountering scepticism would seem to be one of the commonest experiences of allergic people.

This attitude appears to take a number of basic forms. In all of them there seems to be an unwillingness to accept that there is a causal relationship between environmental events and people's symptoms. Thus Roberta N, twenty-five, reported:

My GP is not particularly interested in food allergy and he ruled out the pill as causing my fever and fibrositis. When I was admitted to hospital the various doctors assured me that I was not suffering from any form of allergy and that an allergy would not cause the symptoms I was experiencing.

Roberta's experience of invalidation was typical of sufferers' reports. Judith I's report that when she improved on her elimination diet her GP remarked, 'Could be psychological but if you feel better, carry on,' points to another component of the scepticism evoked by allergy. If a relationship does clearly exist between environmental events and symptoms, then instead of denying the existence of the relationship, the sceptic may resort to explaining it away in terms of 'suggestion' or other psychological factors. Such scepticism is usually automatic and may be termed routine. Perhaps its saddest feature is that those involved often seem to be unaware of the fact that their view represents only one possible construction of the events; they do not even seem to realize that they are being sceptical. Against such unreflective, reflex-like dismissal, sufferers would hardly seem to have a chance.

Automatic or routine scepticism contrasts with what we might call militant scepticism, a position of assumed moral outrage at being asked to consider the possibility that someone might actually be reacting to an environmental precipitant rather than just being 'awkward', difficult', or 'neurotic'. Anna W, aged fifteen, suffers from migraine, as did her paternal grandmother and as does her own mother. One of the precipitants of Anna's headaches is a vanilla-flavoured sweet of the easy-mix variety. Anna's mother described an incident in which her maternal grandmother, who does not suffer from migraine, took them out for a meal at which a vanilla sweet was served. 'Anna ate the vanilla sweet,' her mother reported, 'because Granny was paying for the meal and is extremely hostile to any "allergic nonsense".' She added that, 'the "migraine Granny" would have been rather less hostile'. As this incident suggests, militant scepticism may involve exposing the sufferer to his or her allergens, as if to 'prove' that the whole business is a lot of nonsense. As we saw earlier, Mike P reported that on more that one occasion when he was invited to a meal with friends, he was served peppers without his knowledge, presumably to see if he 'really' got as sick from eating them as he maintained he did. When the predictable reaction ensued, he was angry and his friends were very embarrassed. No similar incidents occurring in medical settings were reported, e.g. deliberate provocation with allergens not done with the sufferer's informed consent as part of a diagnostic exercise, but one respondent did say that her warnings to the consultant about the likely effects of a proposed investigation were brushed aside and when the predictable reaction occurred it was apparently discounted. However, cases of deliberate exposure of allergic people to their allergens by medical personnel who refuse to believe that they are allergic to them are not unknown.

A third variety of scepticism is what we might call open-minded scepticism. This is the case in which the sceptic is aware of being sceptical but is not unduly offensive and righteous about his position. He is willing to listen, at least. Alice A described the reactions of some of her colleagues as follows:

> Working in a psychiatric unit for the past twelve years I know and am known by a number of psychiatrists and other medical staff, with many of whom I have discussed this. Some are very interested, others I feel are not impressed.

The open-minded sceptics offer the allergic a more hopeful social prognosis than any of the others. If they listen, there is a chance that they will hear enough to persuade them to discard their prejudice, though this outcome is by no means guaranteed. Betty S, for example, wrote: 'Most people are sceptical at first but always show an interest – then are either convinced or think I'm "odd".' Rita M told a similar story:

> At first I did not have difficulty, but learnt not to mention it to some people. It has helped that people I know have seen me 'return from the dead', as they put it, since I have held to my 'funny foods'.

Her account suggests that one way that scepticism is overcome is for sceptics to be in a position to observe the effects of a successful elimination diet on someone they know. The mother of Ben C, whose story we heard about at the beginning, also wrote along similar lines:

> Some who have seen the difference think *perhaps* food might be the cause. Others are sceptical. Teacher at school noticed an improvement and co-operated by informing us of 'bad days' to see if these were tied up with diet.

Another deterrent to scepticism is the belated realization that the sceptic is himself affected by allergy. Claire N answered the question as follows:

> No, they have been totally lacking in understanding, particularly my husband, who has ridiculed treatment, etc. but recently his doctor told him that his skin trouble was allergic so he has become more co-operative.

Megan T also remarked that 'some are interested, feeling that the same thing could be their personal problem.'

The three types of scepticism can perhaps best be thought of as points along a continuum with militant scepticism at one end, then automatic or routine scepticism, followed by open-minded scepticism, and finally, at the far extreme, tolerance, acceptance, understanding and sympathy. This account would be incomplete if the positive end of the distribution went unmentioned. Although such reports were less frequent, some respondents did mention that they encountered people who were receptive, supportive and kind when it came to their special problems. Elise O, forty-five, for example, wrote:

> People have been wonderful. Family and friends have happily prepared meals that I can eat and have shown great interest – and great joy at my improvement.

Jennifer H, sixty-one, spoke in a similar tone:

> My husband and family have been exceptionally understanding, helpful and co-operative. Most friends are understanding when the position is explained. My GP is sympathetic and interested. Nurses are usually interested and hostesses helpful, also waiters.

She added the comment we saw earlier about only meeting with scepticism from a few consultants, but these gentlemen are clearly the exception in her exceptional experience. Esther W, sixty-three, also remarked: 'Most people are very sympathetic and understanding. I have had no unpleasant reactions from anyone.' But she, too, added a coda; 'My husband gets fed up when I'm ill so often, but I understand the problem.'

What factors enable people to make themselves understood to non-affected others? Eileen J, seventy, indicated one possible reason for her relative lack of difficulty:

Not much misunderstanding. Since I retired four years ago there have been few occasions for it. Also I can be quite definite in explaining if necessary and this helps. The problem and its remedy are quite clear-cut.

If a sufferer's problem is relatively clear-cut – for example, migraine caused by the usual foods – outsiders will have heard of similar things before and will, accordingly, be better able to assimilate this new instance to their existing schema than if they had only just heard of it and had no schema to which to relate the new findings. But if the sufferer's problem is enormously complex, like that of the multi-allergic Joan P, reception is hampered by lack of anything meaningful to which to relate the new information. Joan wrote of others' reactions to her: 'Nearly everyone has, or has a relative with, some form of allergy, but they find it hard to relate to my extreme reactions.' Her remedy is also complex – desensitizing drops, air purifiers, a hypo-allergenic household, and numerous restrictions on what visitors may do, such as no smoking, no perfumes or hair sprays, etc. – and her reactions may also be acute and near life-threatening. People whose concept of 'allergy' runs to strawberry rashes, hay fever and bloating of the lips after shellfish will have nothing in their previous experience that might enable them to grasp the full implication of a multi-allergic person's condition.

Respondents' reports suggested that it is the practical implications of having an allergic state rather than the mere fact of its existence which people find most difficult to grasp. Sixteen year-old Paula S, who suffers from allergy to grains and a number of other foods and chemicals, contrasted the scepticism of the medical profession with the receptiveness of her peers:

> . . . most people my own age understand and accept it. Most people are interested and ask me questions about it. The only problem is that people do not realize quite how many foods I have to cut out of my diet.

Her report tallies with Elizabeth T's account. Elizabeth, fifty, said that what she tended to encounter socially was 'not misunderstandings so much as a lack of knowledge on the subject'. Denise R also answered the question in terms of other people's knowledgeability: 'Some have vague or no ideas. A few are informed. Orthodox practitioners are normally ignorant and don't want to know or bother as time consuming.' As her comment suggests, the complexity of the subject of environmental hypersensitivity is obviously a deterrent to understanding on the part of people who are not affected. As Margaret L wrote of the problem; 'One has to live with it to really understand.'

To summarize the results of the first analysis of social reactions, we may say that sufferers' predominant experience is of feeling misunderstood by most of the people they encounter, particularly medical and paramedical professionals. Misunderstanding on the part of others arises from a number of factors: the complexity of allergy/hypersensitivity and its practical everyday implications; ignorance and, more importantly, prejudice. In particular, sufferers often report that the rejection they encounter takes the form of stigmatization, mainly psychopathological. They are either overtly labelled or silently regarded as 'odd', 'neurotic', 'hypochondriacal', and so forth. Almost any label in the psychiatric lexicon can be applied, and most of them are from time to time. Those who do not get pseudodiagnostic labels get called 'attention-seeking', 'faddy', 'mad', or other more colloquial variants. In the next section, we will examine this tendency to dispose of what cannot be understood by recourse to derogatory labelling.

Name Calling as a Means of Invalidating Allergic People
This analysis is probably the most revealing about the social position of allergic people. All terms and labels which respondents mentioned in relation to themselves or to other allergic people were extracted from all contexts in which they were used throughout the questionnaire. A grand total of forty-nine different labels was found. They were mentioned by fifty-

nine of the eighty-five respondents, a rate of 69.41 percent or nearly three quarters of the sample. Because some respondents mentioned more than one label, as we saw in the excerpts quoted earlier, the total number of instances of labelling was 108, which represented a rate of 1.27 labels per person for the whole sample. Upon inspection, the terms appeared to fall under four broad headings, as presented in Table 45.

Table 45:   Derogatory labels mentioned by respondents

Psychopathology	*Eccentricity*	*Antisociality*
Neurotic (5)	Fussy (26)	Nuisance (4)
'All in the mind' (5)	Queer (3)	Antisocial (2)
Hypochondriac (3)	Eccentric (3)	Naughty (2)
Anorexic (2)	Cranky (3)	Badly behaved (1)
Nut cases (2)	Health nut (3)	Unsocial (1)
'Psychological' (2)	Odd (3)	Drunk (1)
'Imagination' (2)	Faddy (2)	Awkward (1)
Fragile (2)	Different (2)	
Overanxious (1)	Fanatic (1)	*Condescension*
Overprotective (1)	'Like I had 4 heads'	
	(1)	A bore (2)
Obsessional (1)	Peculiar (1)	Nonsense (2)
Paranoid (1)	Health-food nut (1)	Silly (1)
Mad (1)	Finicky (1)	'Poor thing' (1)
Loopy (1)	Food faddist (1)	Exaggerating (1)
Manic-depressive (1)	Strange (1)	Tiresome (1)
Psychopath (1)		'Reasonably normal'
		(1)
'Stoned out of my		
mind' (1)		
'Round the bend' (1)		
An idiot (1)		
Craving for attention		
(1)		

The table shows that the largest group of terms – a total of twenty – falls under the heading of Psychopathology. In view of the high rate of 'mental' symptoms reported by the group, this finding may not be entirely surprising. Eccentricity, the next largest category, contains only fifteen items, but one of them – the term 'fussy' – was mentioned more often than any of the others, a total of twenty-six times.

The frequent mention of 'fussy' was undoubtedly due to the

fact that the term was itself used in one of the items on the questionnaire:

> Do you find you need to seek extra information about new situations before you feel safe in going into them as a result of having these problems? What sort of information do you feel you want or need to know? Do others seem to appreciate your concern or do they regard you as 'fussy' (or some other such thing)?

Reg R gave one typical response to this question: 'I am always considered fussy and a health-food nut, also a hypochondriac!!' Sarah V gave a more elaborate reply tending towards the same end:

> I need to know about the food supply, whether it is acceptable for me to provide for my own needs, and what is actually available. Family and some friends understand. Most others seem to regard it as faddiness, fussiness, obsessionality or other term of abuse. Doctors other than my own have been unhelpful, sarcastic, arrogant, destructive.

Her response was also typical of the concerns of many fellow sufferers. Andrea A wrote, for example:

> Yes, I have to seek information if I am going anywhere as to what food will be available and what food I can eat. Some people appreciate the situation. Some people think I am fussy or neurotic.

Polly U's report had a different ending:

> I expect everyone regards me as fussy. I am only grateful I have a doctor who understands and treats me with respect and gives me all the help he can.

These reports imply that when others understand the reasons for the affected individual's concern and the damaging consequences of lack of attention to detail in environmental matters, they can appreciate the situation and do not dismiss it with a derisive label. Thus Roberta N emphasized the role of lack of understanding: 'Some people seem to think I am fussy about what I eat and tend not to understand that certain foods make me ill.' In Paula's experience, by contrast: 'People are normally very concerned and once I've explained what happens to me if I do eat things they believe in it and understand why I appear to be fussy.'

But it also seemed that some respondents found trying to explain their predicament very difficult and refrained from doing so, even at the cost of remaining misunderstood. Thus Alan B wrote: 'I don't tell anybody for fear of being branded neurotic and fragile.' Anna W's mother said something very similar: 'I suspect that I would be regarded as *very* fussy if I did enquire about food and drink before going anywhere.' And Dierdre E echoed Alan when she wrote: 'I keep quiet about it, for fear of being classed as fussy.'

Emerging from these reports is one of the most invidious predicaments with which allergic people may be faced. On the one hand, if they tell other people about their special difficulties in the hope of getting them to understand, they run the risk of being labelled and misinterpreted and stigmatized instead. But on the other hand if they *don't* tell other people about their special difficulties, they may run a greater risk of exposure to their allergens and of developing a reaction in public, which is also likely to be misunderstood and lead to labelling and stigmatization. For some sufferers, at least, there seems to be no course of action available that does not entail a risk of major unpleasantness. A further twist to the tail of this dilemma is that both the sufferer's symptoms and the regimen he or she must adopt in order to avoid the allergens that provoke them can be made the basis for stigmatization. Thus in some contexts the sufferer will be regarded as a nutter if he/she displays his/her symptoms but also if he/she displays regimen-following behaviour such as enquiring into the constituents of a composite dish that is being served, bring 'safe' food along to a party, or eating foods in a strict rotation. In this condition, there is almost no getting away from being misunderstood and this fact is one of the many environmental irritants that help to undermine the efforts of the afflicted to live normal lives.

Those who have never been in a similar position may wonder what the problem is. Why is it so awful to have other people regard you as 'fussy' or whatever, that you would rather run the risk of making yourself sick than to enquire whether the sauce has any of your pet allergens in it? Aren't these people really just making mountains out of molehills?

The answer is, of course, a resounding 'No'. Being thought 'fussy' or worse is only the tip of a very large iceberg and the real trouble lies in the assumptions that accompany such labels. Like an onion, this problem has many layers. First, people who are regarded as in any way 'different' or 'odd' tend not to be taken seriously as the rest of us who are not. It is a well-known observation in hospitals that the patient's credibility is automatically in doubt by virtue of the fact of being a patient. In hospital case notes, the patient's statements are transcribed in inverted commas and the staff often seem to develop the habit of mentally adding inverted commas around everything the patient says even in conversation that isn't written down. Those who find this difficult to believe should either ask any recent in-patient or, better still, get admitted somewhere for endocrine investigations themselves. But the same process of bracketing off the statements of those who seem 'odd' also occurs widely in everyday life. We are all familiar with such phrases as, 'Oh, don't mind him/her; he/she's a bit peculiar.' Even if people don't come right out and say it, it is often clearly inferrable from their behaviour *vis-à-vis* others whom they regard as 'different' that the thought has not failed to cross their minds. It is very difficult to survive socially if everyone tends to discount what you say.

Secondly, people who are not taken as seriously tend to be avoided, possibly for fear of 'contamination'. A kind of cryptic infectious disease model would appear to underlie much common social behaviour in relation to those who are 'different'. Proverbs capture this mentality in well-known words: 'Birds of a feather flock together'; 'A man is known by the company he keeps' and others of this ilk. It is extremely difficult to survive socially if no one seems to want to know you.

Third, those who are regarded as 'different' begin to find that they are at an extra disadvantage when competing in the open market for opportunities leading to a share in the world's goodies, whether educational or occupational. One sour or equivocal phrase, more innuendo than anything else, inscribed in a letter of reference or, more likely, reported informally over the telephone, can seemingly finish an applicant's chances. And just as nothing succeeds like success, so nothing seems to breed subsequent failure so much as past failure. This social disadvantage is in addition to the numerous physical disadvantages we discussed in the previous chapter. It is also found in other social situations: residential accommodation, social service provisions, in fact almost anything involving environmental exposure. It is virtually impossible to survive socially if no one will educate, employ, house, or look after you.

Fourth, the effect of this erosion of social credibility and goodwill on many sufferers is to lower confidence and self-esteem even more, which also does not help their chances for social survival. It is totally impossible to survive socially if you've been made to feel you've got to apologize for your very existence.

These disadvantages are in addition to the risk of being made sick when others discount a sufferer's report that certain foods or substances can have adverse effects and expose him/her, whether inadvertently or deliberately, to an allergen. They are also in addition to the damage that may be done if the person is subjected to routine institutional processing as if the psychopathological attribution were true. They are also in addition to the practical, economic, social and psychological costs of all the opportunities lost over the years because of the original problem, which may contribute directly or indirectly to the person's condition of social anomaly. Thus being regarded as 'fussy' or some other such thing is only a stone cast into the social pool. The nasty ripples of implication can spread to all corners of social life and to physical functioning as well. There is a lot more to this name-calling than initially meets the eye.

The findings about social reactions to allergic people suggest that particularly for those who are moderately or severely affected by allergy, both the condition itself and their obligatory regimens of self-management may contribute to, or indeed may constitute, a form of social deviance, which we may follow the sociologist Edwin Lemert in defining as 'violations of norms or departures from social expectancies'[10]. The norms thus violated may be either subtle or obvious and they are multiple: eating what is offered and clearing your plate; having a drink like everyone else; joining in; and not objecting to other people's habits, pets, washing powder, upholstery, cooking utensils, hair-spray, cosmetics, etc.; not displaying symptoms or symptomatic behaviour; not cancelling arrangements at the last moment; not asking for special treatment or special food; not questioning minutely what everything contains; not seeking advance information about eating arrangements, heating arrangements, air conditioning, the presence of animals, houseplants, smoke, etc.; not being in wildly different states at different times, and so on. If such expectations can be said to hold in the world at large, they are all the more binding in medical settings where, above all, patients are meant to be seen and not heard. In short, people in our society, especially when they are patients, are *commonly expected to behave as though they were not allergic* and, as with any form of social deviance, those who are not able to conform to the rules tend to be blamed for their inability to do so by those who can.

The result of this state of affairs is often an increase in the burden of distress their condition already entails and an amplification of their already considerable secondary handicaps. Thus as a result of a physical anomaly, the sufferer may find that he/she has also become a social freak. It appears from the motley collection of labels respondents mentioned that allergic people do not constitute a clearly defined social category in their own right but instead are assimilated in the public mind to a number of pre-existing deviance categories: the mad, the odd, the bad and the sad. Whatever names they are called, the name-calling serves to situate them beyond the pale of the normal social order. For some, the constant misunderstanding and lack of sympathy are as difficult to live with as their underlying biological handicap. As one allergy victim said to me once in conversation, 'This illness doesn't kill you, but sometimes it can make you wish you were dead.'

Social death can be just as real, and sometimes more painful, than its biological counterpart. It takes longer and the victim remains aware of what is happening and the comparison between what is and what might have been remains as omnipresent as it is invidious.

Short of full-scale social extinction, the sufferer may experience a host of special worries as a result of the condition. We shall turn to these in the following chapter.

9.

Special Worries of Allergic People

Earlier on I argued that everyday social situations might come to acquire special new meanings for at least some allergic people who, because of their sensitivities, encountered unusual difficulties in relation to them. In this chapter we will examine the results of an enquiry into this interesting question of how a biological anomaly transforms the victim's social perception. Respondents were asked:

> Are there any situations that worry you more than they might worry someone else who didn't have these sorts of problems? If so, what are these?

Their answers to this question will lead us further into an understanding of the nature of their predicament.

Worrying Situations

A breakdown of the different broad categories of situations mentioned is given in Table 46. The headings in the table and their general order of frequency show a strong similarity to the information collected in answer to the question on limitations and provide corroboration of the earlier findings. It will now be useful if we look at the kinds of worries these situations provoke.

It is hardly surprising that people who have problems with common foods should feel ill at ease at the prospect of social eating/drinking situations in particular or social situations in

Table 46:   Situations causing special worry

Situation	Responses		Respondents	
	n	%	n	%
Social eating and drinking	49	21.59	24	28.24
Social situations–general	42	18.50	31	36.47
Contact with medical services	38	16.74	16	18.82
Travelling	23	10.13	14	16.47
Physical and environmental factors	22	9.69	16	18.82
Ensuring treatment	16	7.05	8	9.41
Allergy: symptoms and effects	12	5.29	11	12.94
Work	12	5.29	5	5.88
Family concerns	11	4.85	7	8.24
All situations	2	0.83	2	2.35
None/don't know/no reply	13	—	13	15.29

general, because so much of social life centres on communal eating. But what was problematical in these situations was less the food itself than social pressure to consume it. Harry L, fifty-nine, wrote, 'I worry about being pressurized to drink whisky and beer like the others.' Jenny M, now in her mid-twenties, reported that she had once had a similar problem:

> Not any more but I used to find it very hard saying 'no' if someone I didn't know very well made me a cup of tea/coffee as a favour without asking me first, as I didn't want to offend them. Hence I often used to make myself ill.

Rachel N also wrote of her worry about 'parties and pubs where one is pressurized'. Pat Z referred to 'occasions where drinks are being handed around. It's not always possible to get a ''soft'' one without prolonged explanations.' Others worried about social events where 'food made in their honour' would be served, because it would be difficult not to consume it but also difficult to do so, and explanations of their dilemma would not be what was on the agenda.

For many respondents, having to explain one's special difficulties was a source of extra worry. Many expressed reluctance to reveal their condition to others, for fear of being misunderstood and rejected. Veronica S wrote of her fifteen-year-old son, Edward:

Ed spent nearly a week with his aunt earlier this month. It helped him to see that he could cope in someone else's house who was understanding, but we still have a big 'block' over going to, say, camp or abroad with people whom he doesn't want to tell.

Other mothers also said that their afflicted children often didn't want other people to know about their dietary problems because they hated to feel 'different'. For adults, the problem seemed to be more a matter of etiquette. Sue M said that 'visiting people for the first time for a meal' was difficult for her because she felt awkward about having to ask for special consideration and equally uncomfortable about trusting to luck. Louise P echoed her sentiment; she worried about 'going to dinner at people's I don't know well and can't remind beforehand'. In some cases these difficulties led people to refuse invitations to dine out; others attended but brought their own safe food along.

In addition to being pressurized to join in and having to explain why they couldn't, respondents also spoke of worrying about the presence of a number of physical factors in environments where they might enter. Here the problem was not so much pressure to participate as the inescapability of the noxious substances once they had entered into the situation. Amongst the substances and objects mentioned were paraffin stoves, the heating in conference halls, overheated, hot, stuffy rooms, bonfires, smoke, flashing lights, perfumes, hair-sprays, mentholated rubs for rheumatic complaints, tobacco smoke, traffic exhaust fumes, gas radiators, and other noxious inhalants. Respondents' reports suggested that these sorts of troublemakers were often both more difficult to avoid and the source of problems that were more difficult to explain than food reactions. People who react adversely to foods can deal with their hypersensitivity by choosing not to eat food set before them, by selecting plain foods, bringing their own along, or declining invitations to eat out. They have a great deal of choice, in most ordinary social situations, about whether or not they eat things that are likely to disagree with them. They can also anticipate which occasions are likely to involve food and can take certain precautions such as forewarning the hostess or restaurant in advance, bringing their own reserve supply of safe food 'just in case', or wearing a Medic-Alert bracelet. Moreover, if they try to explain their problems to other people, there is a chance that they will encounter some, although as we saw by no means universal, understanding. In the present climate of opinion, food allergy is coming to be accepted as a more or less 'normal', if terribly inconvenient, problem.

Inhalant sensitivity differs from food sensitivity in most respects. Whereas food and drink are voluntarily consumed and can thus be voluntarily avoided, inhalant exposure, particularly in an indoor setting, may have already taken place by the time the victim becomes aware of it; it may already be too late to prevent damage occurring. The same can also happen in outdoor settings, for example when a car is stuck in traffic behind a diesel vehicle. Or, as Randolph has shown,[1] the inhalant may be borne by air from great distances towards the hapless victim. Whereas food-sensitive folk can always resort to bringing their own or having it brought in, it is well-nigh impossible for the inhalant sensitive to carry their own envelope of uncontaminated air along with them on social occasions, though some are able to acquire oxygen apparatus to revive themselves after exposures. Moreover, it is often difficult to get people to accept explanations of the problem of chemical hypersensitivity or sensitivity to organic inhalants which takes other forms than the conventional respiratory symptoms (particularly CNS symptoms), because most people have no prior acquaintance with such manifestations and hence no conception that they are possible. If others are to understand, the sufferer must educate them himself in the implications for dealing with him. This task is made more difficult by the fact that the effect of inhalant, and particularly chemical, hypersensitivity is often to incapacitate the victim, so that once exposure has occurred the hapless sufferer may be in no position either to explain what has happened or to retain credibility if he tries. Finally, whereas refraining from a food makes no demands on those who are able to consume it, refraining from chemical exposure may mean that the sufferer has to ask others to refrain from such preferred behaviours as smoking, wearing perfume, after-shave, or hair-spray, etc. in their presence. In certain situations this may be impossible, so the situation must be avoided in order to be safe.

The reports of the chemically sensitive members of the sample had a characteristic flavour which reflects these differences between food and chemical problems. Doreen W, fifty-eight, who reacts adversely both to foods and chemical and organic inhalants, wrote:

Unable to travel on trains, buses, because of perfumes and smoke. Unable to go in our church hall as it has gas radiators that smell. Also getting in church and finding that someone sitting near me is smelling of perfumes and various rubs people use for rheumatism, etc. I've had to get up and out quickly as the urge to faint is so bad. I'm now getting scared to go anywhere that I cannot get away from quickly. I would never dare to travel in a coach where I was trapped.

Doreen was not the only one. Clarissa D, sixty-nine, who reacts adversely to numerous chemicals as well as foods, wrote, 'Yes. One dreads going on a coach, in case of hair-spray, after-shave, etc.' Paula S, sixteen, who is pursuing school examinations in biology and chemistry, reacts with confusion, weepiness, fatigue and headaches to ethanol. She said that she experiences special worries 'in a laboratory when I am not sure which chemicals have been used in the lesson before'. Like Sue M, the egg-sensitive lady who needed to know whether an egg had been anywhere near a saucepan in which her meal had been cooked, and Ted J, the asthmatic student, who needed to know whether a cat had previously been in a room in which he was going to sleep, Paula needs to concern herself with potentially troublesome *historical* features of situations she enters as well as with their actual present state. It takes little imagination to appreciate how readily such concerns might be misinterpreted by people who didn't understand the problem.

Not only the past but also the future could be problematical for some respondents. Several people reported worrying about the state they would be in at any given point in future. Brian G described his problems as follows:

At work, planning ahead, particularly meetings, is difficult due to not being able to cope when the time comes. (After a few hours at work I frequently have to return home to bed.) I always have to brief someone else who more often than not has to take over. Meetings that go on after normal hours demand reserves that I haven't got. Overtime is out of the question . . . .

We should recall that Sarah V, in answer to the question on limitations, also mentioned staying late at work as a problem for her. Brian's other problem, 'planning ahead', was also mentioned by Pamela C, a fifty-seven-year-old retailer who suffers from migraine. Pamela said that 'arrangements made in advance' cause her particular worry, for the same reason as Brian. And we may recall, too, from the discussion of limitations, the worry of Helen F, another migraineur, about 'never being sure of being able to keep a date and having to decline taking on responsibilities for fear of letting people down'. From these reports it is clear that sufferers find the unpredictability of their own state a special worry which people who do not suffer from intermittent paroxysmal disability or chronic low fatigue threshold do not have to contend with.

In addition to its worrisome unpredictability, sufferers had other concerns arising from their allergic condition. In some cases, their special reactivity put them at potential risk of physical danger. Thus Reg R noted that 'water irritation effects make muscles twitch and worry me when driving or working machinery after washing or bathing'. Barbara G expressed a fear of learning to drive: 'I'm not frightened of actually driving,' she said, 'but of the depersonalization which happens and in this situation is dangerous.' Others courted risk of social embarrassment. Claire N spoke of worry about 'the heating in conference halls – probably due to the lack of negative ions. I fall asleep however interesting the subject.' Denise R mentioned 'situations in which I need to be alert and look my best' as especially worrisome because her numerous allergies often left her feeling half-doped and looking terrible. In a somewhat different vein, Polly U described another of the many vicious circles which seem to characterize the experience of so many allergic people.

> *All situations* worry me more than the average person and this is yet another factor which lowers my allergy tolerance level. However, as one of my main symptoms is 'stress', this becomes a 'chicken and egg' situation.

And in a single chilling statement, Marge E described the innermost fear of fellow-sufferers whose allergies seem to be spreading to more and more substances: 'I am worried that I may become allergic to all foods.' Thus for some allergic people the condition itself can create hazards to safety, efficiency, stress tolerance, and even survival. Worries about these possibilities are an added burden that must be lived with.

For others, the condition spreads its malign influence by economic means. Thus Bernice W answered the special worries question as follows:

Almost everything, I should think. I have no money, not enough to live on, really. I do not think I can leave the children to their own devices, so can only take part-time jobs if I can get them and one just cannot earn sufficient from a part-time job.

As we saw in the chapter on limitations, others in the survey sample shared the problem of limited ability to work, so Bernice is probably not the only victim with the perpetual financial worries she describes.

Money is not the only commodity the supply of which creates worries for allergic people. Rita M indicated another area of difficulty: 'Sometimes I cannot get some of the things I need due to drivers' strikes, etc. and I realize how dependent I am on "special foods".' Although it is entirely understandable, this problem would not be likely to occur to people who can simply pop along to the supermarket and fill a trolley, even less so to people whose idea of being unable to obtain special foods means that their car has packed up ten miles from the nearest Macdonalds'. People who become irate when ambulance drivers go on strike would probably not blink on hearing that the wholefood shop delivery van drivers had done likewise. But for the sufferer for whom the 'Big Mac' and most of the chemicalized contents of the supermarkets are 'off limits', the problem of food supply can be terribly important. As we shall see in the following section, this problem is particularly acute when sufferers become patients in hospital.

Contact with Medical Services

One of the most important findings of the survey was the high proportion of respondents – nearly one in five – who said that they worried about what would befall them if they came into further contact with medical services. Although several recent authors such as Cousins[2], Weitz[3] and Millman[4] have described some of the outstanding health hazards to the general public which today's hypertechnical and impersonal health services entail, as yet no one seems to have explored the particular risks

to which allergic people may be subjected in their contacts wit
doctors, hospitals and other paramedical personnel.

Table 47:   Aspects of contact with medical services causing speci:
worry

Category	No. of responses
Hospitalization–general	9
Possible drug reactions*	6
Hospital food	5
Reactions of hospital staff	4
Being ill–general	4
Accident or emergency	3
Facing unknown GP	1
Being ill abroad	1
Dental treatment	1
Medical investigations	1
Hospital water	1
Deprivation of nutritional supplements	1

*Includes drugs, binder in tablets, antibiotics, anaesthetics

The particular features of medical situations whicl
respondents said they worried about are shown in Table 47. I
is clear from the list that these people are worried abou
situations that are realistically possible and in which the threa
of exposure to their allergens is quite objective. They are no
envincing 'hypochondriacal' or 'neurotic' worries about :
collection of fanciful catastrophes but realistic, adaptive anxiet·
which appears to be proportional to the degree of exposure risl
and of the improbability that in all but the most enlightenec
settings their legitimate concerns would be acknowledged
understood, and dealt with effectively and humanely.

Sarah V gave a multifaceted answer to the question whicl
deserves our scrutiny:

Admission to hospital – terrifying thought. Might be wors·
than the disease. I would worry about not being able to ge
safe food in hospital and being misunderstood by staff if :
showed concern about it. If I got hungry enough to eat dice·
food and had a reaction, I'd worry that no one would know i
was a reaction or what to do about it. Also, I doubt whethe:
they'd let me carry on with my vitamin and minera
supplements. Being deprived of them would make me mor·

sensitive to allergens, so I'd be more likely to get ill. Investigations would be worrying since they may involve ingesting things. In my experience, no one wants to know if you warn them it could make you sick. The whole scene would be a total nightmare.

These themes, with the exception of her point about the vitamins, cropped up again and again in others' reports. Andrea A echoes many of Sarah's sentiments:

If I had to go into hospital the food problem would worry me. Also if they gave me any tablets, antibiotics, or anaesthetics which I may be allergic to. I would also worry about the reaction to my problems of the doctors and nurses.
I also have to have extensive dental treatment soon and I am worried about the effect of that.

Barbara G gave her reply in schematic form but the message was the same:

Hospital treatment:
a) Allergy to drugs, etc.
b) Allergy to food.
More people would have to know about my problems.

For Betty S the whole topic was quite unthinkable:

I worry occasionally about the prospect of illness and my possible reactions to drugs. In case of an accident – I just won't think.

The founders of the National Health Service would probably be most unhappy to think that prospective patients might find the prospect completely unthinkable, but they do – and not without reason.

Besides the omnipresent threat of exposure to allergens, respondents also mentioned with trepidation the prospect of being misunderstood. Christina T, for instance, wrote of 'fear of going to hospital, where no one would understand'. Rita M was concerned about making herself understood: 'I'm afraid of an accident and not being able to explain that I am allergic to so many things.' Dominique D, by contrast, emphasized the risk of psychopathological stigmatization. Her worry concerned 'the inevitable contact with the medical profession and resulting implication that it's "all in the mind" '. And Diane G reported:

> The only problem I can see would be if I were to have to stay in hospital for any reason, as I found the reactions of all rheumatic specialists to be absolute disbelief that my condition could be caused by an allergic reaction and this has been repeatedly 'pooh-poohed' as nonsense.

It is sad to think that so many people must apparently learn to expect and accept this sort of dismissive reception as a matter of course. In view of the present state of medical enlightenment, however, it is hardly surprising. What is surprising is only that more respondents didn't say the same.

However, the fact that so many respondents did express worry about going into hospital suggests that their previous experiences of hospital life have not given them much confidence in the ability of routine institutional care to deal with their non-routine sorts of problems. Sue M's report of her stay in hospital seems to confirm this suggestion. Sue wrote:

> I was in hospital once and I was specifically asked if I had any allergies. I told them and it was duly written down – and completely ignored. Every meal seemed to be made with egg and as I was not given an alternative choice I had to do without.

It is not difficult to see how frustrating and demoralizing this sort of experience could be. Anyone to whom it happened might well begin to wonder what was the point of asking in the first place if the information wasn't going to be acted upon. This situation could readily engender a sense of powerlessness, which is a feeling known not to be especially conducive to the maintenance and recovery of health. Add inadequate nutrition at a time of unusual stress and you have a recipe for making people worse rather than better. The cumulative effect of being haplessly on the receiving end of such blatant shortcomings in health-care provision can be the definitive loss of any residual confidence in the ability of those in charge to deliver the benefits which are implicitly promised in exchange for the sufferer's submission to the patient role. If in addition the 'care' is dispensed with bad grace – such as Alan B described when he said he had been 'treated as an absolute nuisance' when in hospital with an unrelated complaint – it can readily seem like an utter travesty of what health-care is meant to be.

Of course, such experiences do not befall all allergic people. Some, we recall, reported having met with nothing but kindness and understanding from those in charge of looking after them in hospital. But they do seem to occur to quite a number of those who cannot simply accept foods and other substances without question just because it is expected of them to do so. The relative prevalence of dissatisfaction with being cared for in hospital can be gauged from the frequency with which respondents reported resorting to more obviously beneficial forms of outside help. But even here problems can arise, as Jennifer H explained:

> I am naturally concerned should any emergency arise, e.g. I be rushed to hospital after an accident or for any other cause – having to contend with problems of food and water.
> There could be a financial problem of obtaining treatment, which is not available on NHS or BUPA.
> One's life-line hangs by a thin thread, there being so few doctors practising the desensitizing treatment. If one had to move to another area, it could be very difficult to get treatment.

Whichever way we look at it, the fact of possessing an allergically reactive constitution creates special worries for sufferers in relation to their medical experience. Whether they worry about what would happen if they did come into medical contact or about what would happen to them if they were deprived of contact, they seem to encounter problems which derive from the basic fact that the system is simply not geared to dealing with their special needs.

To some allergic people, hospital care undergoes the same sort of grotesque transformation as the rest of social life. They do not see going into hospital primarily as an opportunity to be helped but rather as an occasion to be maligned, damaged, left to go hungry, and even persecuted. For this reason, many become understandably reluctant to seek medical attention for other independent conditions for which effective help is potentially available because seeking this help would mean running the risk of exposure to an otherwise thoroughly frightening and dangerous situation. These people's perception of medical settings as hazardous to their health is not a distorted paranoid vision. In many cases it represents a veridical perception of the way things are, namely, inimical to environmentally vulnerable people and impervious to their needs.

The National Health Service is based on catering for those to whom the infectious disease and sudden trauma models of illness are relevant. At all levels, from the smoke-filled waiting rooms in casualty departments to the chemical-filled corridors of the wards to the mass-produced high-allergen menus and medications dispensed on them, the modern hospital provides environments of maximal inappropriateness to the care and feeding of allergic people. Nor are hospitals alone in failing to make provision for those who suffer from intolerance to the twentieth century: almost all public eating facilities without exception share the same basic ethos of mass production and massive pollution – which may be why it is so difficult for hospital patients to get people there to acknowledge their need to avoid these environmental hazards. The hazards are regarded as normal and those who object to them are seen as abnormal, with all that that entails, if they object.

In view of the degree to which the presence of their allergens is taken for granted in today's society, it is not surprising that allergic people have their special worries. What is surprising is that their entirely legitimate and adaptive concerns with avoiding them are so often misconstrued as evidence of maladaptive behaviour. This misconstruction is one of the many paradoxes of their condition.

The unfortunate situation in which so many allergic people find themselves will not quietly disappear if other people pretend it isn't happening. As more and more people develop unusual reactivities to the unusual new substances in our crazy environment and discover that these sensitivities are the cause of mysterious illnesses that creep up on them, it will become increasingly necessary that provisions be made to deal with them. In the following chapter, we will look at the survey group's constructive suggestions for doing something about the present unsatisfactory state of affairs.

10.

What Is to be Done?
Sufferers' Views on
Needed Social Changes

No account of a complex socio-medical problem would be complete if it did not include some indication of what form possible solutions might take. The question in such cases is whose views should be taken into account. What normally seems to happen is that once the problem is brought to official attention – usually as a result of some disgraceful incident that hits the front page of the national dailies – a panel of professional 'experts' is appointed. This panel then sits in learned and protracted debate, without being able to agree on basic principles and definitions, let alone anything else. Meanwhile the problem continues to fester much as it did before it became an official issue – which, sad to say, seems to be the point of the exercise.

The stagnation that occurs in the corridors of official expertise does not, however, prevent ferments of constructive activity arising amongst the grassroots. The reason for this unofficial problem-solving activity is that people, being the curious creatures they are, perversely refuse to desist from suffering just because the causes from which they suffer have not received the blessing of official recognition: people persistently died of pneumonia for many years before the pneumococcus was discovered, and the same principle holds for nasty new diseases of civilization such as chemical hypersensitivity and intolerance for foods resulting from modern unnatural eating habits. And since, being the oddities they are, most people if given the choice would prefer not to suffer unnecessarily, sufferers from many unofficial conditions are often highly motivated to find ways of ending their suffering. Therefore it can often be assumed that victims of a problematical condition will of necessity be better informed about the nature of the problem to be solved, more highly motivated to find a solution, and more imaginative in their efforts to do so than the average gaggle of academic elder statesmen who are on the spot because they just happen to be good at committees.

Ecological problems are a field in which this tendency to delegate responsibility for finding a solution to precisely those people with the least idea of what they are about is particularly marked. In the past few years, popular understanding of environmental intolerance has outstripped that of the majority of doctors – clinical ecologists and orthomolecular physicians and psychiatrists being about the sole exception to this dismal generalization. American clinical ecologist William Philpott has aptly characterized this state of affairs:

> Some medical professionals are in the dilemma of waiting for five-year double-blind studies of 100 cases which then have to be confirmed by two other independent five-year double-blind studies before they will venture even a feeble spark of recognition about that which the public considers already to be common knowledge.[1]

Almost the only matter about which the establishment 'experts' seem to be able to agree is that under no circumstances are the views of the afflicted to be taken seriously. This viewpoint is understandable in terms of the acknowledged necessity of maintaining the status quo at all costs. If the aim of official policy is to ensure that things remain as they are, then the very last thing to do is to canvass the opinions of those most likely to object.

In view of these considerations, which some who have not recently had face-to-face contact with the system may find unduly cynical, the approach adopted in the present study may appear as anything from mildly to moderately subversive. My own view – on the basis of the findings so far, acquaintance with many sufferers from ecological disorders, and much contact with the system – is that it is not unreasonable to suggest that the only true experts about the social problems of living with ecological disorders are the people who, willy-nilly, do so every day of their lives, namely, the victims themselves. The officially acknowledged 'experts', who so frequently distinguish themselves only by the depths of their ignorance, could not realistically be counted on for an edifying account of sufferers' everyday problems because their predominant response to these is to deny steadfastly that they exist outside the sufferer's imagination. I would therefore argue that the best way of getting sensible ideas about what ought to be done to improve the lot of sufferers is to ask them directly for their views. Accordingly, survey participants were asked the following question:

> Can you think of anything that might be done to make these sorts of situations less worrying or difficult for people with these sorts of problems?

In our discussion of their answers to this question, we will consider suggestions according to broad band widths of frequency with which they were given.

Most Common Suggestions

The three most common suggestions offered by respondents are presented in Table 48, and show that sufferers are fully aware of the nature of the social problems they are up against. In the minds of the greatest number of respondents, the foremost needs are for greater awareness on the part of the general public, the medical profession and other professionals, and for the means through which enlightenment can be effected.

From the prevalence of these responses, we may infer an underlying model of social change in the mind of group members. The group's astuteness is evident in their emphasis on the prime importance of social understanding as a pre-

Table 48:   Suggestions made by between eighteen and twenty-nine respondents

Suggestion	f
More publicity in the media	29
Greater public understanding and sympathy	21
Education of doctors and other professionals	18

requisite for social action. The group realizes that unless other people know about the problems they face, no action is likely to be taken to make things better. The model seems to assume that other improvements will follow from an increase in general understanding, but the group's prior experience of the beneficial effects of recent media coverage provides a reasonable basis for such an assumption. As Rita M commented:

> . . . the more people realize the effects certain things have on our body they will have more compassion. I think this is already happening.

We saw in a previous chapter that a number of respondents reported a change in public tolerance in the wake of the allergy publicity campaign in Britain in the late 1970s and early 1980s. These reports, and the many mentions of 'scepticism' which we examined, suggest that those who have most to gain from the 'allergy is not all in the mind' paradigm shift are conscious of the fact that it is under way and keenly attentive to any signs of its progress. Helen F also wrote that what would help was 'publicity, which I think is happening for all illnesses, physical and mental'. Thus the group would seem to possess a very sophisticated level of historical consciousness. The study does not yield any evidence to suggest that the reactionary opposition shares this awareness of the ongoing revolution in sensibility that is occurring.

Respondents singled out a number of different aspects of this revolution for comment. Some, like Rita, emphasized the importance of people coming to appreciate the consequences to the sufferer of allergen exposure. Thus Rachel N remarked that what was needed was 'even more publicity about allergies and the dangers of eating the wrong food'. Sue M suggested 'letting people know how ill people with allergies can become'. Others emphasized the social benefits that might ensue. Margaret L remarked that 'a lot more publicity to explain allergies in magazines might help others to be more understanding'. Yvonne J said she would like to see 'more discussion on television and in magazines, etc. so that unaffected people can appreciate the problems and make allowances'. And Michael S added, 'More knowledge would make people more understanding and enable them to help themselves and others.' There was widespread agreement with Elizabeth T that 'it would help if the general public knew more about allergy and its effects, so that they would understand better'. But some, expressing their view in wistfully personal tones, suggested how far there is still to go in the revolution. Heather C, mother of two-year-old hyperactive Jason undoubtedly also spoke for many when she said, 'I wish people could understand about food allergies and I wish that I had more support and understanding.'

Other respondents spelled out the specific nature of changes in public understanding that they would wish to see. Roberta N, for example wrote: 'There should be more sympathy with people who have these problems, especially food allergies, as people tend to think you are antisocial at times.' Sylvia K gave a similar comment: 'More education and general acceptance that it's OK to refuse things because of sensitivities to them and that this doesn't mean one is rejecting the situation or the person offering them.'

Such changes would obviously make it easier for allergic people by relieving some of the invidious pressure to conform to what everyone else is doing, even at risk of being made ill. Taking a somewhat different tack, Anna W's mother said she would like to see the prevalence of allergic conditions acknowledged:

Better publicity and education. Most people think it's only a tiny minority. I suspect it's not so tiny.

Once people realize that allergy can mean them, too, they are likely to be more sympathetic to their fellow-sufferers. In all these cases, respondents seemed to wish, most basically, that others could view the situation in such a way as to replace them within the normal social order.

When commenting on the potential benefits of greater enlightenment amongst professionals, respondents hinted in their replies at an underlying model of decentralization of knowledge and expertise similar to the one I put forward earlier. According to this model, knowledge about allergy and hypersensitivity and ways of managing these conditions are too important to be regarded as the exclusive prerogative of the medical profession. Instead, they should be disseminated amongst health, social service and educational professionals at all levels throughout the social system. Thus Sarah V said that what she thought would help was 'education of the general public, doctors and paramedical staff including nurses, hospital dietitians and caterers'. Mothers of hyperactive children homed in on teachers and health visitors. Ruth M, the mother of Lee, an eight-year-old hyperactive boy, is a contact for one of the branches of the Hyperactive Children's Support Group. In her answer to the question, she noted:

> Education seems to be the main worry of parents who contact me. I feel teachers should be made aware of the problems these children face daily. Also Health Visitors could play a bigger role if they were enlightened.

Twelve-year-old Prudence P's mother made a similar observation: 'I think all health visitors and teachers should be more aware of the possibility of food allergy and how it can affect babies and young children.'

Not surprisingly, those in contact with providers of adult services focused their comments on these. Catherine H's husband, for example, wrote:

> Yes, education of doctors, psychiatrists, and the public at large. A few doctors who have longstanding problems due to food allergies are usually good converts.

His comments on the interest expressed by doctors who know from their own experience what allergy can do is reminiscent of Claire N's report on her husband's change of heart when he came to realize that he, too, was affected. Other respondents mentioned GPs, hospital doctors, and hospital staff generally. Joan P, afflicted with total allergy, was outspoken in describing the outcome of medical re-education which she felt was needed: '. . . doctors should be trained or retrained to recognize people with allergies and understand clinical ecology and not treat us like nut cases.' Doreen W echoed her sentiments: 'Educate doctors and people that this is a real complaint and we are not all nut cases.' In their comments on doctors, as in their comments on the general public, respondents aimed at normalization of the condition.

However, the group was divided in its views on the appropriate way for their condition to be regarded. On the one hand, as we have seen, some respondents wished the public to made aware just how sick hypersensitive people can become if exposed to their allergens, so that others should be better able to understand the lengths that affected people may go to in order to avoid exposure. Kate F, who proposed that the condition should be called by a name other than 'allergy' so that 'it could be looked on as a genuine illness or something like that' was another respondent who wanted the condition to be legitimized by reference to the debilitation, disability and distress it can cause. But on the other hand, some respondents proposed that these untoward reactions should be regarded as essentially normal phenomena. Thus Hazel S remarked: 'Only through the media and educating the general public not to look upon this as a sickness can we hope to achieve any results.' And Betty S expressed the view that it would be helpful 'if food allergy [were] recognized as a major modern cause for illness and accepted as normal'.

At first glance, it might appear as though respondents wanted things both ways. But if we consider that they are actually using the concept of 'normality' in several different senses, pathological and statistical, the confusion disappears.

In referring to the untoward effects of allergy that they would like other people to appreciate more, respondents use the concept of 'normality' in the sense of an absence of pathology. In this sense, allergy is clearly abnormal – people who suffer from it deviate, often significantly, from the norms of health. But what they are saying when they suggest how useful it would be for others to regard this pathology as 'normal' is that, given the joint occurrence of a highly allergic constitution and a highly allergenic environment, illness is, in a statistical sense, an expectable, average, or 'normal' occurrence: under the given circumstances, it represents the most probable outcome, just as getting wet represents the most probable outcome of falling into a lake. It would be quite *ab*normal if this did not occur. Moreover, from Anna's mother's comment that the proportion of the population that is affected is probably 'not so tiny' as official estimates would make it out to be, it seems that another meaning of 'normality' has crept in.

In this sense 'normality' is that which is found in the majority of the population, whether or not it is 'normal' in the pathological sense, and the degenerative diseases of affluence that increasingly afflict the middle-aged and elderly in Western society are 'normal' because most of the population have one or other of them. Far from adopting a contradictory position that can easily be shot down, the group shows a sophisticated awareness of the complexity of the whole concept of 'normality' which is to be admired for its comprehensiveness rather than decried for its flimsiness. Joan's lament about her fellow-sufferers being dismissed as 'nut cases' by doctors suggests the direction in which any accusations of intellectual shoddiness might more appropriately be directed.

Somewhat Less Common Suggestions

Suggestions that were given by between six and twelve respondents are shown in Table 49. These ten suggestions appear to represent beneficial social developments that might be expected to occur as a result of more enlightened attitudes on the part of the general public and service professionals.

Table 49:   Suggestions made by between six and twelve respondents

Suggestion	f
Improved food and product labelling	12
Help from GP for sufferers	12
Provision of appropriate services in NHS	11
Increased availability of safe foods and products	10
Better medical attitudes to sufferers	10
Better diagnostic and treatment methods	10
Official recognition of the condition	8
Research into causes and effects of allergy	8
Wider availability of information for sufferers	7
Government ban on dangerous products and substances	6

These suggestions show, once again, that sufferers are aware of the complexity of the problems they face. The changes they would like to see include alterations in regulations governing the use of hazardous substances, labelling of permitted products, an increase in the range and availability of hypo-allergenic and otherwise 'safe' products, massive alterations in NHS provisions for allergic people, and acquisition and dissemination of information relevant to the condition. Let us examine some of their recommendations in greater detail.

In order to make the environment both safer and more predictable, respondents proposed legislation regarding the use of additives in foods and the indication of their presence on product labels, a ban on lead in petrol and dangerous wrappings such as clingfilm on foods. Labelling of food products with full

particulars of all ingredients was understandably widely recommended. Suggestions included the specification of whether the
'sugar' in a product was derived from cane or beet, of the exact
type(s) of 'vegetable oil' or 'food starch', detailed, labelled
menus in restaurants, listing of excipients in medications, and
full information on the contents of mixtures to be consumed for
hospital investigations. The feeling behind these suggestions
seemed to be that the consumer has a right to know what he/she
is getting and that manufacturers and others who withhold this
essential information are putting many people at unnecessary
risk of untoward reactions.

As for increasing the range of 'safe' products, recommendations included making available products free from MSG and
other additives, offering a special range of chemical-free products in major food chain-stores, having fresh, natural, uncontaminated foods available in public eating places, clinical
ecology shops, shops stocking gluten-free foods and other
similar products, and making available in Britain a wider range
of hypo-allergenic products which are manufactured in the
United States and described in American clinical ecology
books. Information sheets concerning 'where to buy' were also
put forward as potentially quite useful.

The most revolutionary suggestions pertained to medical services for sufferers. They deserve our particular attention.
General practitioners were widely regarded as having an important role to play in diagnosis and treatment of food allergies,
both as providers of primary care and as collaborators with the
more specialized practitioners. Generally speaking, GPs, along
with the specialists, were regarded as not being very 'receptive
or interested' (Bernice W). Several respondents described additional difficulties arising through the failure of their GPs to provide what treatment they could. Brian G, for example, said that
he courted problems at work because of having to take time off
to attend a clinical ecology clinic for treatment. His very
understanding employers allowed him uncertificated sick leave
to attend the clinic;

> So far I have managed to get through without an absence of
> three days, which would need a medical certificate, but this
> would be a problem, since I was not referred by my GP to the
> clinic. Presumably the only answer is co-operation between
> GPs and the few doctors who carry out this type of allergy
> treatment.

Brian is not the only respondent who has problems because of not having been referred to the clinical ecologist by his GP. We may recall Rosina K's report of worrying that her GP might 'cross us off his list because we chose another way'. Other respondents complained that their GPs were reluctant to prescribe for them. Andrea A said that what she thought would help was:

. . . far more understanding and belief on the part of doctors to accept this illness and to give medication when needed. There is a drug called Nalcrom which blocks allergies and which I have asked my doctor to prescribe for me, *strictly for social functions*, but he refuses to do so.

In an earlier chapter we recall that Paul R complained that his doctor withheld medication until he was 'very ill indeed'. Sue M complained of being treated with amusement instead of adrenaline in a casualty department when she appeared in the throes of a bad reaction. And Sarah V reported that although her GP had got as far as writing to the manufacturer of Nalcrom for prescribing information, he had 'baulked at prescribing it', even just to find out whether it would work for her. We recall, too, that many others were assured that they would 'just have to learn to live with it' since 'nothing could be done about' their problem. 'I can't believe there is so little that can be done,' commented Sue M, who works in a medical library.

If help for their troubles was not forthcoming from their GPs, many respondents felt it ought to be available elsewhere in the NHS. Dierdre E said that what would help was 'clinics to help sort out food problems. For people like me,' she added, 'pills, tablets, and potions are not the answer.' Catherine H's husband expressed the view that 'incorporation of alternative medicine within the NHS' was necessary, adding that, 'this will come, I am sure, for acupuncture'. Nell F emphasized that the facilities would ideally have to be ecological: 'an environmentally safe place where one could be sorted out, as in the USA' was her eminently sensible recommendation for improving the lot of sufferers. At the very least, Diane G remarked, 'many more clinics such as the one in Basingstoke, set up all over the UK' would undoubtedly help. And Doreen W emphasized the cost to sufferers of the absence of such provisions: 'Get the NHS to do something as seeking help privately costs so much money.'

But services were not the only improvement in medical provisions that respondents felt was needed, without a great improvement in medical attitudes to sufferers and more sympathetic and constructive behaviour towards them, the proposed new facilities might not be very much less damaging than the present lack of them. Kate F complained that what was required was:

. . . more help and understanding from NHS doctors, hospitals, etc. I had nothing but insults from them when young and no help now.

Elizabeth T also expressed annoyance at the behaviour of doctors:

It amazes me that so little is known about these kinds of allergies, particularly by the medical profession and their scepticism makes me very cross. Of course, I realize that they have not the time to listen to us, but if only they did I am convinced they would free themselves of a large percentage of their regular patients – and what an improvement this would be in the general workforce of the country.

Elizabeth's comment implies that improving the present unsatisfactory state of affairs does not in the first instance necessarily imply a host of costly new resources but rather a more efficient and humane deployment of resources that already exist. Most doctors are not physically hard of hearing, but many felt their doctors either did not seem to know how to use their ears or wish to be bothered. Several respondents, Helena Y ('Yes, get hospital doctors to listen to patients,') and Sarah V ('doctors listening to patients') felt that simply listening to what patients had to say would go a long way towards helping. But listening by itself was not enough. It would also help, Sarah continued, if there were 'less scorn and derision from doctors' and 'less willingness to dismiss allergic patients as "neurotic", etc.' In a similar vein, Diane G said she would like to see 'more understanding or at least consideration by these specialists that [an allergic basis to sufferers' symptoms] might be a possibility'. And Andrew F said that for some sufferers 'psychiatric treatment for symptoms might help', but that unfortunately there was still a stigma attached. These comments make it clear that improvement of the psychosocial and interpersonal aspects of health care were high on the group's list of priorities and an important precondition to effective institutional change.

Official recognition of the condition by the medical profession as a whole was another heartfelt need. Joan P, the severe multi-allergic, recommended that 'the BMA should recognize this illness'. Without official recognition, changes in provisions were not likely to be forthcoming. Eleanor B shared Joan's view. 'It would be nice,' she wrote, 'if the illness could become recognised and if the medical profession could help more.' Jennifer H echoed the recommendation of 'acceptance by the medical profession and NHS of the condition'. And Sally C spoke of how valuable it would be if there were 'a willingness on the part of GPs and of the rest of the medical profession to accept and put into practice the clinical implications of allergy'. It is truly remarkable that people whose lives can be as disrupted by their illness as our respondents' lives have been by their allergies should have to feel that they are suffering from a cause of morbidity which is not officially considered to exist.

In view of the lack of status which their condition has been accorded, it is not in the least surprising that respondents should regard the development of better methods for diagnosis and treatment as an important priority. They seem to appreciate the occult fact that doctors are happier to diagnose conditions for which an objective 'test' exists, preferably one for which they can sign a slip and send the patient elsewhere to undergo. In the present state of what passes for knowledge, they also seem on the whole to be happier about treating conditions for which specific medications can be prescribed, particularly if assays exist for monitoring their levels in the body. Whether we like technological medicine or not, doctors often seem to thrive on it, and our astute respondents appear to realize that if they wish to elicit the help they need their condition had better be able to lend itself to processing in the medically preferred manner.

Thus respondents' suggestions included the 'development of better diagnostic tools for detecting allergies' (Sally C); making advice more readily available to sufferers 'to enable them to work out what causes their allergies and providing support whilst getting them under control' (Alice A); 'help to find substances causing the condition' (Christina T), and GPs 'helping patients through the investigations'. On the treatment side, they called for 'a total cure' (Henry J); 'better antidotes' (Paul R); 'more information and specific knowledge of what will help fast' (Beverley C); 'ways of building up general health' (Polly U); 'reduction of the side-effects of steroids' (Virginia H); 'methods of restoring damage that foods have done' (Catherine H's husband), and 'research into vaccines to help people become tolerant to the foods they react to' (Veronica S). In a similar vein, Eileen J wrote, 'If a harmless and effective vaccine or inhalant that didn't cost the earth could be made available, it would be a blessing to people with multiple allergies.'[2] Collectively, respondents emphasized availability and safety and wished to see remedies that either prevented symptoms developing in the first place or undid damage that had already occurred.

Respondents were well aware that such developments would require research and called for it with enthusiasm:

More research. (Paul R; Sue M)

I think it's time the medical profession did very much more research into loss of sense of smell and taste. (Pat Z)

More research into causes and effects of allergy. (Sally C)

Research and more awareness of what we are doing to our beautiful world with pollution. (Joan P)

Perhaps if a single root cause . . . were to be established, then a simple or single remedy could be made available. (Eileen J)

Commenting on the questionnaire itself, Irene H expressed her approval: 'Research like yours excellent,' she wrote.

Less Common Suggestions

Suggestions made by between two and five respondents are shown in Table 50. These suggestions seem to refer to grassroots-type efforts to live efficiently with the condition oneself and to reduce unnecessary difficulties for others. They are largely self-explanatory, but we may look briefly at suggestions for banning common allergens in public places. Janet I, for example, a chemical victim, called for 'no-smoking rule in

Table 50:   Suggestions made by between two and five respondents

Suggestion	f
Prudent living	5
Detect and avoid offending substances	4
Labelled menus in restaurants	4
Reduction of allergens in public places	4
Hostesses enquiring about guests' allergies	3
Being offered choice of foods	2
Self-help groups	2

restaurants, no smoking or smoking in one room only at parties, better ventilation or smoking-room rule in pubs – also no dogs'. Theresa K, by contrast, said she didn't feel people could be induced to 'stop smoking or wearing strong-smelling perfumes, lacquers, etc.'. The difficulty she anticipates was touched upon earlier in our discussion of some of the differences between food and chemical intolerance, namely that with foods it is only the sufferer him/herself who has to refrain but with chemicals others are also affected.

Suggestions Made by Single Individuals

In addition to the consensual suggestions we have already looked at, individual members of the group mentioned a number of other things that could not be readily coded under the previous headings. They are shown in Table 51 and are a mixed bag of items, ranging from wearing an identification disc to facilitate proper treatment in case of emergency, through government action regarding the location of major sources of environmental pollution, to faith in God. We have already examined the suggestion that the condition be called by a name other than 'allergy'. The only other item that may not be entirely self-

Table 51:   Suggestions made by individual sufferers

Suggestion	f
SOS locket	1
Understanding from employers	1
Name other than 'allergy' for the condition	1
Single person self-catering units	1
Buffet serving	1
Careful siting of factories and refineries	1
Faith in God	1

explanatory is Brian G's point about the importance of understanding from employers. Brian was referring to the fact that his employers tolerate his erratic presence at work. As we saw, he frequently becomes exhausted during the day and has to leave work early. In addition, he is often away from work in order to attend the desensitizing clinic for treatment. He is fortunate that his employers allow him to have these absences as sick leave without a certificate. Others who are not so fortunate encounter many additional difficulties as a result.

The survey group's constructive suggestions for improving the lot of sufferers appear to imply a sequence of events. Stage one is the massive publicity campaign that will lead to such an increase in public understanding and sympathy for the affected that in order not to lose face the medical, paramedical and other service professions will see to it that their members become at least as knowledgeable as the laity. In stage two, enlightenment having spread upwards from the grassroots to the medical establishment, tolerance for ecological practitioners within the NHS will improve to the point where they no longer have to fear for their jobs and much-needed services can begin to be provided at the public expense – with considerable long-range savings to the exchequer from the resulting reduction of chronic disease. Meanwhile, significant initiative from the grassroots will continue in the form of lay advice and support services and of the promotion and funding of much-needed research. It seems likely that lay organizations will have to take the lead in starting ecology clinics, since they are more aware of the magnitude and urgency of the need for them than the medical establishment.

Simultaneously, manufacturers will realize the enormous potential market for additive-free and special diet foods and other hypo-allergenic products and will start to produce ranges of items to be sold at competitive prices. As a result of the increasing availability of such products, hospitals and other public-catering facilities will find it increasingly possible to provide safe menus for affected people. Hostesses, similarly, will be better placed to avoid poisoning their allergic guests. As more and more people come to be aware of their own hypersensitivities, social gatherings are likely to become less of an ordeal for the hypersensitive because, increasingly, they will be able to count on finding something they can safely consume and on not being pressurized to overstep their limits for the sake of being sociable. Smokers – if any still exist – will obligingly congregate in one room in order not to pollute everyone's environment.

There will also remain much that individual sufferers can do to help themselves, starting with the detection and avoidance of their culprits, joining self-help groups for advice and support, and organizing their lifestyles in order to avoid exposure to established sources of difficulty and to other sources of pollution that might lead to the development of further problems.

On a higher level, under pressure from grassroots organizations and possibly even from an enlightened professional establishment, the Government will have to bestir itself to take initiative in reducing the overall environmental hazard to actual and potential sufferers: lead in petrol, additives in food, aerosols, tobacco smoke, plastics, and industrial effluents, among other things, will all require attention.

When all is said and done, the ecological casualties of today will no longer find themselves regarded as marginal human beings, because for many years to come they are likely to represent the majority.

11.

Summary and Conclusions

The main findings of the study can be summarized as follows:

1. Allergic people tend to have multiple allergies.
2. There is no one type of allergic person; all kinds of people can have allergies.
3. The majority of allergic people report a positive family history of allergy.
4. An allergic tendency tends to reveal itself before adulthood.
5. Particular manifestations of an individual's allergic tendency may change with time.
6. Women seem to become allergic to a wider range of substances than men.
7. Virtually any bodily, sensory or behavioural system can be affected by allergy.
8. A large proportion of allergic symptoms affect the central nervous system, behaviour and psychological functioning.
9. Women tend to show a wider range of symptoms than men, generally speaking, but they do not show a wider range of psychological symptoms.
10. Foods that are common constituents of diet are more likely than uncommon foods to cause adverse reactions.
11. Cereal grains – especially wheat, milk and dairy produce are probably the most common British food allergens.
12. People who are allergic to foods are more likely than not

to be hypersensitive to chemicals.

13. Our common food allergens are surrounded by an aura of tradition and commercialism which jointly militate against general recognition of their role in disease.

14. Foods, chemicals and other allergens may contribute to the pathogenesis of depression, psychosis, migraine, and childhood hyperactivity. They are also implicated in some cases of anxiety, tension, depersonalization, sleep disturbance, phobias, obsessions, and other psychological disorders.

15. The majority of allergic people seek medical help for their condition at some time in their lives.

16. Most sufferers who see one doctor about their condition eventually see more than one doctor about it.

17. The allergic basis of many people's problems is not often recognized at primary-care level.

18. The allergic basis of many people's problems also escapes detection by many specialists.

19. Conventional medical interventions bring little benefit to the majority of allergic people who undergo them and also carry a relatively high risk of complications.

20. Alternative medicine often seems to be ineffective against allergies but when it is effective it can give much better results than orthodox medicine and also carries less risk to those who undergo it.

21. Clinical-ecology treatment offers a higher rate of benefit and a lower rate of risk than either conventional or orthodox medicine.

22. Allergic people are inclined to go on seeking help until they find something that is helpful.

23. Of necessity, allergic people tend to be extremely active in the management of their own condition. Their self-help efforts compare favourably in outcome with those of the professionals from whom they seek help and carry a much lower risk of unanticipated adverse reactions.

24. Allergic people tend to read about their condition.

25. Allergic people tend to be more knowledgeable about allergy, clinical ecology, alternative medicine and nutrition than most of the doctors they see.

26. Self-help groups in Britain play an important role in advising sufferers from allergic conditions. They provide access to information, books, relevant practitioners,

concrete advice and moral support.

27. Most allergic people are handicapped by their condition in their everyday lives at least to some degree.

28. Many different factors affect the degree to which a person is socially handicapped by an allergic condition.

29. For a proportion of allergic people, normal life is virtually precluded by their condition.

30. Virtually any area of everyday life can be spoiled for some allergic people.

31. Feeling misunderstood, particularly by professionals, is a very common experience of allergic people.

32. On the whole, allergic people perceive lay people as somewhat more likely to misunderstand them than to understand them.

33. On the whole, allergic people perceive professionals as considerably more likely to misunderstand them than to understand them. Thus medical encounters are often both frustrating and unrewarding for allergic people.

34. The more complex an allergic person's condition, the less likely other people are to understand it.

35. The practical implications of the allergic state are what other people find most difficult to comprehend.

36. Encountering scepticism is another very common experience of allergic people.

37. A certain degree of social stigma is attached to being allergic.

38. Allergic people can be stigmatized by others either because of their symptoms or because of their efforts to avoid exposure to their allergens.

39. There is no clear-cut 'allergy' stereotype.

40. Allergic people, when stereotyped, are usually seen as psychopathological, eccentric, antisocial or pitiable.

41. Allergic people are often given pseudodiagnostic, derogatory labels.

42. This name-calling has many potentially harmful social repercussions.

43. People in our society are commonly expected to behave as if they were not allergic.

44. Allergic people have many special worries as a result of their condition. Medical experience is especially worrying to many, especially contact with hospitals. These worries are often misunderstood.

45. Allergic people would like to see more publicity for their condition, leading to greater public sympathy and understanding. Education of professionals, better medical attitudes and services, and government legislation regarding unsafe substances are also high in their list of priorities for improving their lot.

The picture of the situation of allergic people in Britain today that emerges from the findings of the survey is not a pretty one. It suggests that the allergic and hypersensitive are amongst the most neglected groups of sufferers. But whereas in the case of the elderly, the mentally ill and the mentally handicapped, the services – or lack thereof – provided by the State are at least topical issues and the focus of active political disgruntlement, if not always of remedial action, the allergic remain a shadowy and amorphous group stirring at the edges of public awareness. As we saw in the discussion of name-calling, they lack even a popular stereotype of their own. As a socio-medical entity, the allergic do not yet exist.

The fact that their suffering is not widely recognized does not, however, mean that it does not happen. If anything, it means that those who are already moderately to severely handicapped may suffer even more because uncomprehending professionals, instead of offering them help, make light of their difficulties and expect them to go away and do likewise. The shameful neglect that these people experience at the hands of the system responsible for providing for their care is nowhere more apparent than in the unrewarding and unhealthy nature of much of their contact with hospitals where, as we have seen, they are more likely even than in the everyday world to be misunderstood and to have their special needs ignored or misinterpreted.

Although the National Health Service does not provide even a facsimile of effective and efficient care for the majority of allergic people, it has not been notably receptive to those practitioners who might be expected to make a start in this direction. One after another, the majority of medically qualified clinical ecologists practising in this country have had to leave their hospital posts. Those in general practice who are competent to offer clinical ecology services find that they can only do so on a private basis. In his BBC Reith lectures, Ian Kennedy commented on the disparity in access to medical services amongst members of social classes 1 and 2 and classes 4 and 5.[1] Ecological services would seem to exemplify this general situation in a particularly poignant way, since it seems likely that those in the higher social classes are probably able to eat more varied diets and inhabit less chemically contaminated environments and so may be less likely to develop ecological disorders from these causes.

One consequence of the failure of organized medicine to provide much-needed services to the mass of the public is that practitioners who are not medically qualified have stepped into the yawning gap. As we saw in the case of Barbara G, they can get results which are just as good as those obtained by many medically qualified ecologists and considerably better than those which our sample reported to have been obtained by non-ecological doctors. We have also seen that the lay self-help groups get excellent results in many cases for those who turn to them for advice when all the system seems to be able to offer is either reassurance that the child will outgrow his difficulties or prescribe a bottle of tablets so that his mother is less distressed by the chaos the child's disorder brings forth. A number of alternative practitioners are also adopting ecological methods, with beneficial results for their clientele. Like the allergic people they serve and the medically qualified clinical ecologists, these lay practitioners also commonly encounter trouble from the medical establishment. They find themselves globally denounced as 'cranks' by one of its well-known pillars.[2] In one case that has recently been reported,[3] a patient suffering from anxiety, depression and eczema was referred to one of Britain's few NHS-based ecologically-oriented clinical psychologists for attention to her psychological symptoms. Her eczema was concurrently receiving treatment, not very successfully, from a consultant dermatologist. On the dietary regimen devised by the psychologist, the woman's anxiety and depression lifted and her skin also showed a dramatic improvement. But did the consultant dermatologist rejoice in his patient's unexpected recovery? No, instead he threatened the psychologist with dire personal consquences and the patient with withdrawal of his care for the rest of the time the psychologist remained involved in her case. This is probably the worst example of medical chauvinist piggery in the field of inter-disciplinary care of ecological patients, but other incidents could be cited. Another psychologist had a middle-aged man referred to her for attention to his multiple somatic symptoms for which no organic cause had been found after extensive investigations. The man was said to be suffering from 'anxiety' and to be rather 'hypochondriacal'. He had not responded to treatment with tranquillizers and the referring doctor asked whether the psychologist might have some 'suggestions that might lead to symptomatic relief for this man'. The psychologist was unable to understand the man's complaints in psychological terms and proposed a dietary approach to their elucidation and remediation. The referring doctor raised no objection at the time, but after the patient had been seen and told that the sudden abdominal bloating he experienced after meals was probably due to something he had eaten, advised to read the Mackarness paperbacks, and try eliminating certain foods which his diet diary suggested might be causing the trouble, the referring doctor apparently took umbrage and complained about the psychologist to a senior colleague.

From these examples, it seems that some doctors – though by no means all – want it both ways. They either cannot or will not themselves provide the ecological care that these patients need and they seem either unable or unwilling to countenance the fact that members of other professions, or even of the laity, might be both able and willing to do so. The implications of their 'dog in the manger' position is that it is better that sufferers should go on suffering than that they should obtain from other sources the help which doctors themselves refuse to provide. In their scheme of things, medical hegemony would seem to take precedence over patient care. It needs little imagination to see who are the losers as a result of these arrangements.

This unsatisfactory state of affairs should not be allowed to continue. More is at stake than simply the mopping up of the environmental casualties who have already succumbed. They are the vanguard and those who come after them are bound to be both worse affected and more numerous, because the environmental conditions that seem to promote the creation of casualties – exclusive bottle-feeding in infancy, premature introduction of solids, a steady diet of over-refined, chemicalized, processed food, chemically polluted air, wholesale use of pesticides, plastics and other chemicals, and so on – will have hit them earlier and have been in force for a greater proportion of their lives. As Joan P, our total allergic, wrote at the end of her questionnaire, 'I have heard that people like me should be held up as a dreadful warning, like canaries down the pits.' Like the canaries that could be used to warn the miners of dangerous levels of poisonous gases in the mines, the total allergics of today merely have a lower threshold for environmental toxicity than the rest of the population. Their message is the same as the canaries' to the miners: unless we get away from the rising levels of environmental and dietary poisons, the rest of us will begin to succumb too. It is not a question of whether, but of when. And unless there are some dramatic improvements in available services, social conditions and environmental pollution between then and now, we will wake up to find that we have no experts to turn to for advice about what to do for the best, no facilities for treatment, no treatment other than trying as best we can to avoid everything in the environment, no one who still wants to know us, and not even any official acknowledgement that anything is the matter with us that pulling our socks up wouldn't cure.

At the risk of sounding cynical, I would suggest that perhaps the only way the situation of allergic people will gain the widespread publicity it needs is for people in high places to begin to lose their tolerance for the world in which we live. The leading practitioners in the field of clinical ecology have themselves all been victims of ecological disorders and have been able to use their own unfortunate experience to understand and remedy the problems of others. What would greatly help in establishing the validity of ecological suffering in the public mind is for someone widely known and respected as a person of unimpeachable integrity to develop a spectacular ecological disorder with significant central nervous system manifestations and to be helped to resume his or her former position in society by means of an ecological regimen and then to write a full-length account of what the experience was like. In the early part of our century, Clifford Beers did as much for mental illness with his classic account entitled *A Mind that Found Itself*.[4] Many needed reforms followed in the wake of his depiction of the way his breakdown was treated.

Meanwhile, it is to be hoped that this account of the everyday problems of ordinary allergic people will help to kindle a spark of much-needed interest and official recognition and to enable those who are not yet affected to deal more humanely with those who are.

Appendix A

Food Allergy Survey

This survey aims to gather preliminary information about people's experience of food allergies and chemical sensitizations, to find out what people know they are allergic to, what they suspect they are allergic to, what forms their reactions take, and what they have done about these problems. The effects on their lives and the difficulties they encounter as a result of these problems is also of interest.

The questionnaire is anonymous, but it will help in analysing the information if you will indicate your age, sex, and occupation below.

Age _______ Sex _______ Occupation _____________

If there are any other comments on your experience that you would care to make, please feel free to write them on the back or on extra sheets of paper.

May I thank you very much for your help in this survey

____

1.   Are there any foods, drinks, or chemical substances which are either swallowed or inhaled that you are aware of having unpleasant or unusual reactions to? If so, what are they and what are the reactions they provoke? (Please include anything you feel pretty sure about, even if the reaction only occurred once.)

2.   Are there any similar substances which you suspect of causing unpleasant reactions but which you are not entirely sure about? If so, what are they and the reactions you suspect they may be involved in?

3.   Do you ever experience unpleasant symptoms which you suspect may be due to something eaten or to a chemical swallowed or inhaled, but without being sure just what may be causing them and without suspecting anything in particular? If so, what are they?

4.   For how long have you had these sorts of difficulties?

5.   Did they appear to be brought on by anything or did they just seem to develop out of the blue?

6.   Do others in your family experience similar problems? Do any relatives have other sorts of allergies, not related to ingesting substances (e.g. skin rashes when particular substances come into contact with the skin)? Any asthma, hay fever or similar complaints in the family? Migraine?

7.   Have you ever had any of these sorts of difficulties yourself, apart from your food allergies, etc? If so, what were they?

8.   Have your allergic difficulties remained the same or changed since they started, either in that different foods or substances have become involved, ones you were previously sensitive to become 'safe', or different reactions caused?

9.   Have you sought medical attention for these problems? If so, what was done about them by way of investigation and treatment, and how effective was/is the treatment?

10.   What have you done about the problems on your own initiative, without outside help? In particular, have you read anything about them, kept diet records or recorded symptoms, or tried elimination dieting, or any other experiments with food or chemical exposure? Have you tried any self-prescribed remedies you may have heard or read about or worked out for yourself? Have these efforts been a help?

11.   Have you sought help from people other than doctors? If so, who, and with what outcome?

12.   Do you find that people you come into contact with (such as family, friends, relatives, hosts/hostesses/guests, waiters, stewardesses, doctors, nurses, other professionals, etc.) tend to understand these sorts of problems or do you run into misunderstandings?   Have   there   been   any   particularly

outstanding incidents of misunderstanding that stick in your mind?

13.   Do you tend to tell people you have these sorts of problems or to conceal the fact that you've got them? Who do you tell? Who do you not tell?

14.   Do others tell you about their difficulties with food allergies and chemical sensitizations?

15.   Do these problems cause you to limit your activities in any way? If so, how (include avoidance of allergenic substances here, as well as avoidance of situations in which exposure to them might occur).

16.   Are there any situations that worry you more than they might worry someone else who didn't have these sorts of problems? If so, what are these?

17.   Can you think of anything that might be done to make these sorts of situations less worrying or difficult for people with these sorts of problems?

18.   Do you find you need to seek extra information about new situations before you feel safe in going into them as a result of having these problems? What sort of information do you feel

you want or need to know? Do others seem to appreciate your concern or do they regard you as 'fussy' (or some other such thing)?

19.   At a later stage of this research, would you be willing to take part in a personal interview which would go into your experience of these problems in more detail? If so, could you indicate your name, address and a telephone number where you can be reached closer to the time (sometime in 1983). If not, not to worry, I'm grateful for your help with the questionnaire.

Name ____________   Address ____________   Phone______

Again, many thanks.

Vicky Rippere

Appendix B

Practical Advice for Non-sufferers who would Like to Help their Allergic Friends, Relatives and Acquaintances

By now the unaffected reader should be better acquainted with the everyday problems of allergic people and may have started to wonder what he/she can do to show more sympathy, tolerance and helpfulness to his/her afflicted friends.

Since these sterling qualities can really only be shown in relation to particular individuals in particular situations, there can be no absolute, hard and fast rules. Nonetheless, a few general guidelines seem to be possible on the basis of the information collected in the survey.

First, examine your conscience and your stock of pat phrases for any residues of the 'allergy is all in the mind' myth and take care to expunge them. If you are thinking to yourself that your friend is really 'making a fuss over nothing', you will give yourself away as someone who does not understand, no matter what you actually do, and your friend would be forgiven for concluding that you are really rather a hypocrite.

Second, it is essential to *listen to the sufferer* and not automatically discount what he/she says simply because it goes against contemporary dogma about food and chemicals which equates convenience with nutritional value and government approval with safety.

Third, even if the effects the sufferer attributes to the substance in question may seem to you less than life-threatening, do not dismiss them as trivial. They may be the tip of a very large iceberg, which repeated contact with the particular allergen — or any allergen, for that matter — may help to expose. With chemicals, particularly, each additional exposure can whittle away at the body's chemical tolerance. More is at stake than merely avoiding a headache, a crop of blisters or whatever: when total environmental tolerance is eroded, there is no sure way of recovering it. Bear that in mind instead of any dark thoughts of 'exaggeration'.

Fourth, in order to be helpful, you will need to know about the individual's habitual safety precautions and try to co-operate with these as fully as possible, whether this means preparing him/her a safe meal when visiting you, remembering to forego your usual perfume, after-shave, or hair-spray when spending time in his/her presence, or banishing smoking or the family pet to another part of the house.

Fifth, if your allergic acquaintance has to call off an engagement at the last moment because of an unexpected reaction or declines an invitation because it is incompatible with adhering to his/her regimen, you can help by not taking it personally and not assuming automatically that it is 'just an excuse'. Your acquaintance probably feels much worse about it than you do and will not be helped by thinking that you've taken it the wrong way.

Sixth, if your acquaintance is so unfortunate as to land up in hospital for any reason, he or she may appreciate it if you enquire about bringing in a supply of safe food and drink. The help of friends may be the only way the sufferer in hospital will be able to get enough to eat or drink.

Seventh, if you are really interested, it would help to find out more about allergy and chemical hypersensitivity. This is not difficult to do because there is now so much coverage of these topics in the popular media. In fact if one reads anything, it is difficult to avoid coming across information on these topics. But in addition your friends can probably recommend some useful paperbacks and will probably be impressed by your show of interest. Your reading may suggest to you new ways to be of assistance to your friend and it may also raise your suspicion that, like him or her, you are also experiencing problems because of sensitivity to some environmental factor. If so, you may find that your friend can do much to reciprocate your effort to be helpful and in this you will be fortunate because often you will get more sensible advice and information from a knowledgeable sufferer than from your doctor or the specialist to whom he sends you.

As a sufferer yourself, you will come to appreciate better what your friend has been up against and to understand the value of having friends who understand.

Reference Notes

Quotation page

1 Hippocrates (1950) *The Medical Works of Hippocrates* Translated by J. Chadwick and W.N. Mann (Oxford, Blackwell Scientific Publications), pp.179-80
2 Anselm L. Strauss (1975) *Chronic Illness and the Quality of Life* Louis, C.V. Mosby Company) p.vii
3 T.G. Randolph and R.W. Moss (1981) *Allergies: Your Hidden Enemy* (Turnstone Press)

Introduction

1 Vicky Rippere (1981) 'Social and psychological hazards of environmental intolerance' in A. Rees and H. Purcell (Eds) *Disease and the Environment* (Chichester, John Wiley), pp137–145.
2 J.K. Wing (1978) *Reasoning about Madness* (London, Oxford University Press)
3 Vicky Rippere (1981) Hazards to sufferers from food intolerance from medical investigations *Journal of Human Nutrition 34*, 4
4 Sir Kenneth Vickery (1980) in Richard Mackarness *Chemical Victims* (Pan Books) p.xii
5 For a comprehensive discussion, see William Ryan (1976, revised ed.) *Blaming the Victim* (New York, Vintage Books).

6   See Richard Asher (1962) Fashions in Disease *Twentieth Century 172* (1015), 17-20. This article is also a good indicator of the degree of unfashionability of allergy, which Asher presents as rather a laughing-stock:

> The trend in medicine today (as it always has been) is to provide diagnostic tags, special treatments and complete causal explanations for every illness that exists, whether or not anything is known about it. We have allergists and allergic departments although there is very little proof of the allergic origin of any of the diseases they treat. The cause of asthma is unknown, but the comforting idea of finding the one special substance you are sensitive to, and of de-sensitizing yourself to it, is so comforting that it thrives. According to the variety of discomforts to which man is subject, so will be the number of comforters provided for him, and the changing vogue in types of disease will continue for that reason

7   J. Soothill (1980) Elimination diets in childhood *British Medical Journal* i, 401-2. For a reply to this letter, see Vicky Rippere (1980) In defence of 'cranks' *British Medical Journal* i, 795.

8   For an interesting and pertinent discussion, see Carolyn J. Rosenthal, Victor W. Marshall, A.S. Macpherson and Susan E. French (1980) *Nurses, Patients and Families* (London, Croom Helm), Chapter 2, pp.25-50.

Chapter 1: Food Allergy: A personal account

1   This experience is described more fully in: Vicky Rippere (1982) Biochemical Victims: False negative diagnosis through overreliance on laboratory results – a personal report *Medical Hypotheses* [in press].

2   Theron G. Randolph and L.B. Yeager (1949) Corn sugar as an allergen *Annals of Allergy 7,* 651-61

Chapter 2: A Group of People

1   This case is described more fully in: Vicky Rippere (1981) Chemical Victim *Bethlem and Maudsley Gazette* Spring Issue, 23-4.

2   Richard Mackarness (1976) *Not All in the Mind* (London, Pan Books), p.37

3   The occupations were coded according to the official

classification: Office of Population Censuses and Surveys (1970) *Classification of Occupations,* (London, HMSO).

4 J.W. Gerrard, G.C. Ko, P. Vickers and C.D. Gerrard (1976) The familial incidence of allergic disease *Annals of Allergy 36,* 10-15

5 D.P. Cantwell and G. Tarjan (1979) 'Constitutional-organic factors in etiology', in J.D. Noshpitz (Ed) *Basic Handbook of Child Psychiatry* Vol.2, (New York, Basic Books), pp.28-62

Chapter 3: Allergens

1 F. Speer (1970) 'Etiology: Foods' in F. Speer (Ed) *Allergy of the Nervous System* (Springfield, Illinois, Charles C. Thomas), pp.198-209

2 See, for example: R.H. Dreisbach and C. Pfeiffer (1943) Caffeine-withdrawal headache *Journal of Laboratory and Clinical Medicine 28,* 1212-9; J.R. Harrie (1970) Caffeine and headache *Journal of the American Medical Association 213,* 628; B.C. White, C.A. Lincoln, N.W. Pearce, R. Reeb and C. Vaida (1980) Anxiety and muscle tension as consequences of caffeine withdrawal *Science 209,* 1547-8
C.S. Farkas (1979) Caffeine intake and potential effect on health of a segment of northern Canadian indigenous people *International Journal of the Addictions 14,* 27-43
H.A. Reimann (1967) Caffeinism: A cause of long-continued low-grade fever *Journal of the American Medical Association 202,* 131-2
B.D. Ross (1971) Caffeine and fluid retention *Journal of the American Medical Association 218,* 596
J.T. Flynn (1970) Arrhythmias related to coffee and tea *Journal of the American Medical Association 211,* 663
M.C. McManamy and P.G. Schube (1936) Caffeine intoxication. Report of a case the symptoms of which amounted to a psychosis. *New England Journal of Medicine 215,* 616-20; J.F. Greden (1974) Anxiety or caffeinism: A diagnostic dilemma *American Journal of Psychiatry 131,* 1089-92
E.G. Lutz (1978) Restless legs, anxiety and caffeinism *Journal of Clinical Psychiatry 39,* 693-8
T. Colton, R.E. Gosselin and R.P. Smith (1968) The tolerance of coffee drinkers to caffeine *Clinical Pharamacology and Therapeutics 9,* 31-9

A. Goldstein and S. Kaizer (1969) Psychotropic effects of caffeine in man. III. A questionnaire survey of coffee drinking and its effects on a group of housewives. *Clinical Pharmacology and Therapeutics 10,* 477-88

Editorial (1973) Caffeine, coffee and cancer *British Medical Journal* ii, 1031-2

Editorial (1981) Coffee: should we stop drinking it? *Lancet* i, 256

Editorial (1981) Coffee drinking and cancer of the pancreas *British Medical Journal 283,* 628.

R. Vaughan (1981) Coffee in pregnancy *Lancet* i, 554

M.F. Jacobson, A.S. Goldman and R.H. Syme (1981) Coffee and birth defects *Lancet* i, 1415-16

3   See, for example: J.H. van de Kamer, H.A. Weijers and W.K. Dicke (1953) Coeliac Disease. IV. An investigation into the injurious constituents of wheat in connection with their action on patients with coeliac disease. *Acta Paediatrica 42,* 223-31

J.W. Gerrard, C.A.C. Ross and J.M. Smellie (1955) Coeliac Disease. Results of late treatment with gluten-free wheat diet. *Lancet* i, 587-9

J.M. Ruffin, S.M. Kurtz, J.L. Borland Jr, C.R.W. Bain and W.M. Roufail (1964) Gluten-free diet for non-tropical sprue *Journal of the American Medical Association 188,* 162-4

A.B. Arthur, B.E. Clayton, D.G. Cotton, J.W.T. Seakins and J.W. Platt (1966) Importance of disaccharide intolerance in the treatment of coeliac disease *Lancet* i, 172-4

C.C. Booth (1970) The enterocyte in coeliac disease *British Medical Journal 4,* 14-17

Editorial (1970) Coeliac Disease *British Medical Journal 4,* 1-2

R.R.W. Townley and C.M. Anderson (1967) Coeliac Disease. A Review. *Ergebnisse der inneren Medizin und Kinderheilkunde* (N.F. Bd. 26. Berlin, Heidelberg, New York, Springer Verlag), pp.1-44

P.J. Ciclitira, J.O. Hunter and E.S. Lennox (1980) Clinical testing of bread made from nullisomic 6A wheats in coeliac patients *Lancet* ii, 234-6

M. Doherty and R.E. Barry (1981) Gluten-induced mucosal changes in subjects without overt small-bowel disease *Lancet* i, 517-20

4   See, for example: F.C. Dohan (1966) Cereals and schizophrenia: Data and hypothesis *Acta Psychiatrica Scandinavica 42*, 125-52
F.C. Dohan (1969) Is coeliac disease a clue to the pathogenesis of schizophrenia? *Mental Hygiene 53*, 525-9
F.C. Dohan, J.C. Grasberger, F.M. Lovell *et al* (1969) Relapsed schizophrenics: more rapid improvement on a milk- and cereal-free diet *British Journal of Psychiatry 115*, 595-6
F.C. Dohan and J.G. Grasberger (1973) Relapsed schizophrenics: Earlier discharge from the hospital after cereal-free, milk-free diet *American Journal of Psychiatry 130*, 685-8
F.C. Dohan (1980) 'Hypothesis: Genes and neuroactive peptides from foods as cause of schizophrenia' in E. Costa and M. Trabucchi (Eds) *Neural Peptides and Neural Communication* (New York, Raven Press), pp.535-48
M.M. Singh and S.R. Kay (1976) Wheat gluten as a pathogenic factor in schizophrenia *Science 191*, 401-2
J.R. Rice, C.H. Ham and W.E. Gore (1978) Another look at gluten in schizophrenia *American Journal of Psychiatry 135*, 1417-8
5   See Ernest Dichter (1964) *Handbook of Consumer Motivations* The Psychology of the World of Objects (New York, McGraw Hill).

Chapter 4: Symptoms
1   See, for example, Singh and Kay (1976) loc. cit.
D.S. King (1981) Can Allergic Exposure Provoke Psychological Symptoms? A Double-Blind Test *Biological Psychiatry 16*, 3-19
2   See, for example, F. Speer (Ed.) *Allergy of the Nervous System* (Springfield, Illinois, Charles C. Thomas).
W.H. Philpott and D.K. Kalita (1980) *Brain Allergies* The Psycho-Nutrient Connection (New Canaan, Connecticut, Keats Publishing Company)
Theron G. Randolph and Ralph W. Moss (1981) *Allergies: Your Hidden Enemy* (Turnstone Press).
3   W.A. Lishman (1978) *Organic Psychiatry* The Psychological Consequences of Cerebral Disorder (Oxford, Blackwell Scientific Publications)
4   Since writing this section I have learned of the study of

dietary factors in schizophrenia and depression which is being organized by Sanity. The Schizophrenia Association of Great Britain is also involved in a diet study in collaboration with the MRC Environmental Epidemiology Unit at Southampton University.

5   Robert Burton (1972, first published 1621) *The Anatomy of Melancholy* Edited with an introduction by Holbrook Jackson (London, Dent)

6   Editorial (1979) Food allergy *Lancet* i, 249-50

7   Mackarness (1976) op. cit.; Dohan (1966) op. cit.; S.S. Kety (1976) Dietary factors and schizophrenia *Annals of Internal Medicine 84* (6), 745

8   W.A. Hemmings (1978) The entry into the brain of large molecules derived from dietary protein *Proceedings of the Royal Society of London* B, *200*, 175-92

9   C. Zioudrou, R.A. Streaty and W.A. Klee (1979) Opioid peptides derived from food proteins. The exorphins *Journal of Biological Chemistry 254*, 2446-9

10   P.D. Kanof and P. Greengard (1978) Brain histamine receptors as targets for anti-depressant drugs *Nature 272*, 329-33

11   T.N. Thomas and J.W. Zemp (1977) Inhibition of dopamine sensitive adenylate cyclase from rat brain striatal homogenates by ascorbic acid *Journal of Neurochemistry 28*, 663-5

12   D.F. Horrobin and M.S. Manku (1980) Possible role of prostaglandin E1 in the affective disorders and in alcoholism *British Medical Journal ii*, 1363-6

13   R.J. Williams (1956) *Biochemical Individuality* (Austin and London, University of Texas Press).

14   Since this concept does not yet seem to exist, it is probably necessary to invent it. The literature suggests that people differ immunologically in countless ways, from blood group, to particular allergies, to profile of immune globulins, and so forth. It seems likely that individuals will differ in any immunological parameter that is studied. Therefore it seems necessary to assume that, just as people have been found to be biochemically unique, they will also turn out to be immunologically unique.

15   Edda Hanington (1980) Diet and migraine *Journal of Human Nutrition 34*, 175-80

16   Ellen C.G. Grant (1980) Food allergies and migraine *Lancet* i, 966-9

17 See, for example: E.J. Mikkelsen (1978) Caffeine and schizophrenia *Journal of Clinical Psychiatry* 39, 732-6
D.K. Winstead (1976) Coffee consumption among psychiatric inpatients *American Journal of Psychiatry* 133, 1447-50
B. De Freitas and G. Schwartz (1979) Effects of caffeine in chronic psychiatric patients *American Journal of Psychiatry* 136, 1337-8

18 See, for example: W.E. Beebe and O.W. Wendell (1973) 'Preliminary observations of altered carbohydrate metabolism in psychiatric patients' in D. Hawkins and L. Pauling (Eds *Orthomolecular Psychiatry* (San Francisco, W.H. Freeman), pp.434-51

19 B. Feingold (1968) Hyperkinesis and learning disabilities linked to the ingestion of artificial food colours and flavours *Journal of Learning Disabilities* 9, 19-27
B. Feingold (1975) *Why Your Child is Hyperactive* (New York, Random House).

20 See, for example, L.K. Salzman (1976) Allergy testing, psychological testing and dietary treatment for the hyperactive child syndrome *Medical Journal of Australia* 2, 248-51
E.C. Hughes, L. Oettinger, F. Johnson and G.H. Gottschalk (1979) Case report: A chemically defined diet in diagnosis and management of food sensitivity in minimal brain dysfunction *Annals of Allergy* 42, 174-6
F.J. Kittler and D.G. Baldwin (1970) The role of allergic factors in the child with minimal brain dysfunction *Annals of Allergy* 28, 203-6
H. Tryphonas and R. Trites (1979) Food allergy in children with hyperactivity learning disabilities and/or minimal brain dysfunction *Annals of Allergy* 42, 22-7
F.J. Kittler (1970) 'The effect of allergy on children with minimal brain damage' in F. Speer (Ed) op. cit., pp.122-33
J.M. Weiss and H.S. Kaufman (1971) A subtle organic component in some cases of mental illness. A preliminary report of cases *Archives of General Psychiatry* 25, 74-8
For a review of work in the area, see: J.W.T. Dickerson and F. Pepler (1980) Diet and hyperactivity *Journal of Human Nutrition* 34, 167-74

21 M. Mandell and L.W. Scanlon (1979) *Dr Mandell's Five-*

Day Allergy Relief System (New York, Pocket Books), pp.179-92

22 Robert Forman (1979) *How to Control Your Allergies* (New York, Larchmont Books), p.133

23 For a discussion of this point, see: Vicky Rippere (1981) Placebo-controlled tests of chemical food additives: are they valid? *Medical Hypotheses 7,* 819-823.

24 See Irene Colquhoun and Sally Bunday (1981) A lack of essential fatty acids as a possible cause of hyperactivity in children *Medical Hypotheses 7,* 673-9

25 Oliver Gillie (1981) Ssch: This food dye is staying hush-hush *Sunday Times* 14 June

26 See, for example: A.R. Lucas and M. Weiss (1971) Methylphenidate hallucinosis *Journal of the American Medical Association 217,* 1079-81

D. Safer, R. Allen and E. Barr (1972) Depression of growth in hyperactive children on stimulant drugs *New England Journal of Medicine 287,* 217-20

M.B. Denckla, J.R. Bemporad and M.C. MacKay (1976) Tics following methylphenidate administration. A report of twenty cases. *Journal of the American Medical Association 235,* 1349-51

R.H. Mattson and J.R. Calverley (1968) Dextroamphetamine-sulfate induced dyskinesias *Journal of the American Medical Association 204,* 108-10

Q. Case and J.B. McAndrew (1974) Dexedrine dyskinesia. An unusual iatrogenic tic. *Clinical Pediatrics 13,* 69-72

Chapter 5: Help-Seeking

 1 J.B. Miller (1972) *Food allergy provocative testing and injection therapy* (Springfield, Illinois, Charles C. Thomas)

 2 Rippere (1981) *Journal of Human Nutrition* loc. cit.

 3 A.F. Coca (1978) *The Pulse Test: Easy Allergy Detection* (New York, Arco Publishing Company)

 4 For a discussion of the administrative chaos surrounding hyperactive children in Britain, see Steven Box's prefatory chapter in Peter Schrag and Diane Divoky (1981) *The Myth of the Hyperactive Child and Other Means of Child Control* (Harmondsworth, Penguin), pp.7-30

Chapter 6: Self-Help

1 The method and the theory behind it are described in:
H.G. Clark and T.G. Randolph (1950) The Acid-Anoxia-Endocrine Theory of Allergy *Journal of Laboratory and Clincal Medicine 36*, 811-12.
H.G. Clark and T.G. Randolph (1950) The Clinical Application of the Acid-Anoxia-Endocrine Theory of Allergy. *Journal of Laboratory and Clinical Medicine, 36*, 811. For a more recent discussion, see: T.G. Randolph (1976) 'The Enzymatic, Acid, Hypoxia, Endocrine Concept of Allergic Inflammation' in L.D. Dickey (Ed.) *Clinical Ecology* (Springfield, Illinois, Charles C. Thomas), pp.577-96

2 Vicky Rippere (1974) *Antidepressive Behaviour* Unpublished M.Phil. dissertation, University of London
Vicky Rippere (1976) Antidepressive behaviour – a preliminary report *Behaviour Research and Therapy 14*, 289-99

3 W.G. Crook (1977) *Can Your Child Read? Is He Hyperactive?* (Jackson, Tennessee, Professional Books)

4 David Robinson and Stuart Henry (1977) *Self-help and Health: Mutual aid for modern problems* (London, Martin Robertson) pp.52 ff

Chapter 8: Social Reactions to Allergic People

1 The best example of work in this area is probably Jum C. Nunnally Jr.'s study (1961) *Popular Conceptions of Mental Health: Their Development and Change* (New York, Holt, Rinehart and Winston) which deals with mental illness.

2 In his Introduction to *Allergies: Your Hidden Enemy* (Randolph and Moss, op. cit.) Ralph W. Moss makes a similar point:

> Many of a doctor's patients come with multiple symptoms, both physical and mental. Doctors are often taught in medical school that the more symptoms a patient has, the less credence should be given to any one of them, since it is assumed that many such patients are hypochondriacs and have imagined their symptoms. Randolph taught the opposite: the more symptoms a patient has, the more likely he is to be suffering from an environmentally induced disease (p.8).

> Many multisymptomatic people can testify from their own experience that this new lesson would bring benefit to

many if it were to be more widely disseminated in Britain.
3   Thomas Kuhn (1962) *The Structure of Scientific Revolutions* (Chicago and London, University of Chicago Press)
4   Vicky Rippere (1981) *Journal of Human Nutrition* loc. cit. Since this letter appeared I have acquired a client who came to considerable grief during a series of glucose tolerance tests she underwent as an in-patient. Each time she had the glucose, she became uncontrollable and was regarded as 'hysterical' as well as 'difficult'. The possibility that these reactions, which were stereotyped in form, were iatrogenic, was not, of course, considered. On my screening questionnaire for masked food allergy and chemical hypersensitivity, she was positive for corn and other grains. She was very relieved at the suggestion that her 'hysterical' reactions may well have been due to grain sensitivity. It had been a source of considerable distress to her to think that there was something about her psychological make-up that led her to misbehave in situations such as the hospital ward where the investigations were carried out. She is undoubtedly not the only person in such a predicament.
5   See Talcott Parsons (1952) *The Social System* (London, Tavistock Publications) pp.436-9
6   Robinson and Henry (1977) loc. cit.
7   Hippocrates (1950) op. cit., pp.179-93
8   Vickery (1980) loc. cit.
9   Randolph and Moss (1980) op. cit.
10   Edwin M. Lemert (1972, 2nd edition) *Human deviance, social problems and social control* (Englewood Cliffs, New Jersey, Prentice-Hall) p.13

Chapter 9: Special Worries of Allergic People
1   Theron G. Randolph (1962) *Human Ecology and Susceptibility to the Chemical Environment* (Springfield, Illinois, Charles C. Thomas) pp.52-3. See also Randolph and Moss (1980) op. cit., pp.85-6
2   Norman Cousins (1979) *Anatomy of an Illness as Perceived by the Patient* Reflections on Healing and Regeneration (New York, London, W.W. Norton and Company)
3   Martin Weitz (1980) *Health Shock* A guide to ineffective and hazardous medical treatment (Newton Abbot, David and Charles)

4 Marcia Millman (1977) *The Unkindest Cut* Life in the backrooms of medicine (New York, Morrow Quill Paperbacks)

Chapter 10: What is to be done? Sufferers' views on needed social changes
1 W.H. Philpott (1978) 'Ecological aspects of antisocial behaviour' in L. Hippchen (Ed.) *Ecologic-Biochemical Approaches to Treatment of Delinquents and Criminals* (New York, London, Van Nostrand Reinhold) p.117
2 Such a remedy seems to be on its way. See: L.M. McEwen (1975) Enzyme potentiated hyposensitization V. Five case reports of patients with acute food allergy *Annals of Allergy 35,* 98-103

Chapter 11: Summary and Conclusions
1 Ian Kennedy (1981) *The Unmasking of Medicine* (London, George Allen and Unwin) pp.58ff
2 Soothill (1980) loc. cit.
3 Neil Adams (1981) The Case of Anne *Newsletter of the Society for Environmental Theropy 1* (1), 6-7.
4 Clifford W. Beers (1908) *A Mind that Found Itself* An Autobiography (London, Longmans Green)

Useful Address

Action Against Allergy
43 The Downs
London SW 20

British Migraine Association
Evergreen
Ottermead Lane
Ottershaw
Chertsey
Surrey

Chemical Victims
Basingstoke General Hospital
Basingstoke
Hampshire

Food Allergy Association
9 Mill Lane
Shoreham-by-Sea
West Sussex

Hyperactive Children's
Support Group
59 Meadowside
Angmering
Sussex

Sanity
77 Moss Lane
Pinner
Middlesex

Schizophrenia Association of
Great Britain
Tyr Twr
Llanfair Hall
Caernarvon
Gwynedd

Index